T0325127

Therapeutic Communication in Mental Health Nursing

This book introduces an innovative technique for therapeutic communication in mental health nursing, expanding the toolkit for nurses seeking to engage challenging patients who have not responded to more conventional therapeutic methods. Linking nursing communication to current research on metaphor and figuration, it is illustrated with accessible clinical examples.

Metaphor is a key component of talk-based psychotherapies. But many of the patients whom nurses encounter in the inpatient setting are not good candidates for talk-based approaches, at least initially, because they are violent, withdrawn, highly regressed, or otherwise lacking a vocabulary to convey thoughts and feelings. This book offers specific clinical examples of an approach called the "gestural bridge." This is a method for structuring games and physical activities which connect metaphorically to a patient's personal themes, activating narrative and observational agency and enabling an exchange of meaning to begin at a time when conventional language is not available. Rooted in what nursing theorists have called the "embodied" or "aesthetic" way of knowing, this approach is both specific and easily grasped.

Drawing from contemporary work in literary theory, semiotics, metaphor theory, cognitive science, philosophy, linguistics, psychoanalysis, and the arts, *Therapeutic Communication in Mental Health Nursing* is important reading for advanced-level practitioners, students, and researchers interested in communication and relationship-building in nursing.

Shira Birnbaum is a psychiatric nurse, educator, writer, and artist. She graduated from Barnard College, Columbia University, and has worked with chronically and acutely mentally ill adolescents, adults, and homeless in a variety of institutional and outreach settings in the New York and Philadelphia metropolitan areas. She is a project manager at the Brookdale Center for Healthy Aging at Hunter College, City University of New York.

Therapeutic Communication in Mental Health Nursing

Aesthetic and Metaphoric Processes in the Engagement with Challenging Patients

Shira Birnbaum

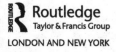

Routledge
Taylor & Francis Group

LONDON AND NEW YORK

First published 2017
by Routledge
2 Park Square, Milton Park, Abingdon, Oxon OX14 4RN

and by Routledge
711 Third Avenue, New York, NY 10017

Routledge is an imprint of the Taylor & Francis Group, an informa business

© 2017 S. Birnbaum

The right of Shira Birnbaum to be identified as author of this work has been asserted by her in accordance with sections 77 and 78 of the Copyright, Designs and Patents Act 1988.

All rights reserved. No part of this book may be reprinted or reproduced or utilised in any form or by any electronic, mechanical, or other means, now known or hereafter invented, including photocopying and recording, or in any information storage or retrieval system, without permission in writing from the publishers.

Trademark notice: Product or corporate names may be trademarks or registered trademarks, and are used only for identification and explanation without intent to infringe.

British Library Cataloguing-in-Publication Data
A catalogue record for this book is available from the British Library

Library of Congress Cataloging in Publication Data
Names: Birnbaum, Shira, 1962– author.
Title: Therapeutic communication in mental health nursing : aesthetic and metaphoric processes in the engagement with challenging patients /
Shira Birnbaum.
Description: Abingdon, Oxon ; New York, NY : Routledge, 2017. |
Includes bibliographical references and index.
Identifiers: LCCN 2016055021| ISBN 9781138244290 (hbk) |
ISBN 9781315276991 (ebk)
Subjects: | MESH: Mental Disorders–nursing | Health Communication–methods | Nonverbal Communication–psychology | Metaphor |
Esthetics | Nurse-Patient Relations
Classification: LCC RC440 | NLM WY 160 | DDC 616.89/0231–dc23
LC record available at https://lccn.loc.gov/2016055021

ISBN: 978-1-138-24429-0 (hbk)
ISBN: 978-1-315-27699-1 (ebk)

Typeset in Times New Roman
by Out of House Publishing

For Helen and Dan

Contents

Acknowledgments

I am thankful to Carolina Antunes and Grace McInnes at Routledge and to Sandra Paul Thomas at the University of Tennessee and *Issues in Mental Health Nursing* for insightful comments on an early version of the manuscript. Maddie Kurtz, Martha Raimon, Kate Dodd, and Paula Radding were patient listeners. I am grateful to Jeff Nurenberg for his exuberance and high expectations, to Mary Kyle for her neighborliness, and to many nurse colleagues over the years, especially Laetitia, Tony, Janet and Cherika, whose unflappable collegiality turned difficult situations into learning. For their support of this and other projects, I thank Geoff Rogers and my other colleagues at the Brookdale Center for Healthy Aging at Hunter College, City University of New York. Steven Schleifer's enduring generosity and insights have enriched my writing and my thinking inestimably. My children Daniel and Helen bring infinite joy to my life and work.

1 Introduction[1]

Sara was one of those remarkable patients, familiar in psychiatric and mental health work, who eats objects that shouldn't be eaten. Batteries, keys, bottle caps, paper clips, knives, nail clippers, Christmas-tree garlands, broken zippers, pencils, chips of plaster and linoleum, coins of all varieties, and all manner, it appeared, of screws, staples, washers, and nails. You could see some of this array in her abdominal X-rays – a radio-opaque detritus from the forest floor of a lived life. Some of these items passed through Sara's digestive tract. Others lingered, necessitating emergency endoscopic procedures or, on multiple occasions, surgery to remove portions of perforated bowel.

A middle-aged, developmentally disabled woman, Sara had been living in a city park and eating from trash cans. Police responded to 911 calls from commuters at a train station where she was found gesturing aggressively and causing a disturbance, and she was taken to a local medical hospital for treatment and evaluation. In the emergency room, radiological scans identified a key, lodged in her esophagus, and dozens of other unusual objects in her stomach and intestines. Multiple endoscopic procedures were performed to clear the gastrointestinal tract, and, once medically stabilized, she was transferred to a nearby psychiatric facility. Over the course of about a month, psychiatrists there sent her out for emergency surgical treatment four more times, X-rays revealing, each time, bizarre new ingestions. A portion of her intestine needed to be surgically removed. From that smaller psychiatric facility, she was delivered, in wrist restraints, to our sprawling admissions department, and, soon thereafter, to one of our general psychiatry units.

At the time we first met her, Sara didn't know her birth name, couldn't give a birth date, and offered no social security number or previous address. She claimed, first, to be 28 years of age. Then 48. Then 31.

She had no known relatives and couldn't remember either parent's first or last name. There were no school records, previous fingerprinting, or other potentially identifying documents. She reported her birthplace as Philadelphia and knew the name Louisiana, claiming to have lived with her mother in the woods there for some period of her childhood. She'd chosen a name for herself with a sound she found pleasing, and, so, Sara is what we called her. During her previous psychiatric hospitalization, she had been diagnosed with schizophrenia, psychotic disorder, foreign-body ingestion, and mild mental retardation. How she'd stayed alive over the years, given the history, we couldn't fathom.

To mitigate the dangers her behavior posed, Sara was placed under a continuous staff surveillance protocol. Legal permission was granted to deny her access to private storage space, clothing with pockets, zippers, buttons, or snaps, eating utensils, and personal possessions such as toothbrushes and combs. She was started on medications to control psychosis and impulsivity. Staff cleaned her teeth by rubbing them with towels and dispensed small quantities of shampoo into her palms when she showered, under supervision. She continued to attempt to grab objects, however, including employee ID badges, pens, syringe covers, and scraps of paper, and she turned aggressive toward the staff attempting to stop her or block her way. She required frequent sedating medication and was moved to a safety room, separated from the general patient areas, after another patient passed near her in a hallway and handed her some coins, which she swallowed. Over the course of the next few weeks, she required multiple additional trips to the emergency room. Her bowel perforated; she became feverish and septic. Multiple surgical procedures again followed, including removal of her gall bladder and portions of her colon. She spent a month in a coma. Then, again medically stabilized, she was returned for psychiatric treatment. This time, there was a medical warning in the chart, with a phone call from one of the surgeons to the hospital medical director: further surgical procedures could not be performed safely. The swallowing had to stop.

On the unit, Sara was bedridden in the beginning, a massive surgical incision bisecting her severely distended abdomen and covered in heavy layers of gauze and tape. We observed her for signs of fever, tended to her wound, and attempted to discourage her from picking and eating the dressings. We confined her to a sparsely furnished room from which all decorative items and trash containers had been removed and door hinges tightly bolted. We counted our supplies – the gauze sponges and tape rolls and gloves and ointment applicators and caps from saline bottles – as if on a surgical unit, so that none of it would wind up in her throat or stomach. We administered enemas to discourage straining and ease the abdominal distension so her surgical wound might heal. We rubbed her skin with lotions to make her more comfortable. A hand-off communication checklist was developed for shift-change, as incoming and outgoing staff together, three times a day, inspected her room for any of the multitude of stray objects that can shake loose from routine hospital procedures. A schedule was established for periodic X-ray evaluations to track her rate of new ingestion.

Foreign-body ingestion, as it is formally known, poses intense and multifaceted management challenges for hospitals and group homes, and there are no therapeutic or pharmacological interventions proven to significantly or durably reduce swallowing behaviors in patients. The behavior is widely documented among the developmentally disabled and well known in borderline personality disorder. Some patients who swallow objects are clearly psychotic or delusional, but many seem remarkably high-functioning, which surprises you when you see them in the throes of an episode – aggressive toward anyone who gets in the way of the compulsion, in that moment, to ingest. It is virtually impossible to build a care environment free of risk, unless you keep someone in shackles, and reports appear frequently in medical and nursing journals lamenting the enormous costs and clinical challenges posed by this elusive, tenaciously complex syndrome. But here was Sara, gracious, friendly, remembering to say "thank you" when served her medications, muttering to herself quietly and glancing into the air, scanning overhead, seeming to be hearing something, with long graceful hands and meticulously clean fingernails, charming in her blue bedroom slippers and floral-print housedress, her hair in neat cornrows, smiling broadly like a jack-o-lantern with her few remaining teeth and asking, politely: if somebody has an MP3 player with speakers, would you mind, please, playing some Bee Gees?

As the weeks passed, Sara's surgical wounds healed, though slowly, as her abdominal distension was not resolving. She began hoisting herself out of bed more frequently, and her confinement began to frustrate her. As her strength returned, so did her aggressive episodes. Staff worried when she began pacing in her room, graduating to slamming herself against walls, rolling on the ground and, within a few weeks, pushing furniture around the floor for hours on end: one day the bed had to be positioned against the wall; the next day, closer to the bathroom door; the day after that, in the corner by the window. The constant motion loosened screws and compromised joints; officers from the Safety department came to inspect, advising a new room-search protocol that included a daily walk-through and visual inspections of all the corners, backs, and undersides of the bed, the dresser, and the side-table, and so on. Sara begged to come out to the shared patient areas, to socialize in the TV room, to sit in the unit porch and throw bread crumbs to the birds outside, to join church services in the hospital chapel and drink coffee at the unit-wide morning meeting. She begged for music, for writing utensils, for art supplies. Increasingly, she needed to be sedated to prevent violent conflicts, as the staff were not authorized to meet these growing demands for independence and activity. The treatment team was stuck. No choice seemed safe. We nurses shook our heads. What is there to do with such a person, who is so utterly likeable and yet so dangerous to her own safety?

To look at the abdominal X-ray of a patient who ingests foreign objects is to feel oneself in the presence of a harvest. It is a harvest of observations, fragments of passing experience, like the collected shards of something barely glimpsed, remembered partially or fleetingly. The paper clip and the crucifix, the wristwatch and the dime, the nametag with the pin on its back – they appear on the screen plate like references loosely connected to one another, as in a collage, insinuating something which might be made coherent, perhaps, if seen some other way; they point to some almost-vanished recollection that might, in time, be retrieved by the mental operation of piecing back together. Every day, one of the hospital staff psychiatrists came to the unit to evaluate Sara. Why, she'd be asked, had she swallowed such-and-such a thing? How did she come to get her hands on it? When was the last time it happened? Is there any intent to do it again? Sara stared blankly at these queries, as if the words themselves mystified. I thought about this at her bedside one morning, perplexed as I sat, wiping her face with a warm washcloth. I had dressed her oozing abdominal wound, wrapping the waste inside-out in a latex glove and encircling it in my palm where she couldn't get a good look at it. I asked the whereabouts of a quarter I knew she'd swallowed some weeks previous. "It's a part of me now," she pronounced, gazing at my face squarely. "No one can take it away."

In nursing school, as in programs for any of the other therapeutic disciplines, we learn that the framing of a question can determine, to a large extent, the quality of the answer. For months, there had been no progress in our understanding of Sara, despite the daily interrogations about why and when and how. But a question about where, suddenly, opened a universe – revealing, remarkably, a grotesque emotional achievement: nameless and without the reference points of home and family and literacy and memory, Sara had turned herself into her own container, a portable corpuscular purse for her own stored data. She had made things "mine," in a sense, by making them "me" – transcending, by way of this unique mental operation, the separation of inside from outside.

The next morning, I woke up early, giving myself time to rummage through my children's bookshelves. I found an old picture book about human anatomy, and I brought it to work, storing it at the nursing station. From that point on, every time I dressed Sara's wounds or administered her medications, I brought the book with me to her bedside, and we sat together to look at the illustrations. This is your digestive tract, I showed her. This is your esophagus. This is your stomach. Here are your intestines. I held her hands over her belly and her chest and her throat, and so on, to show the locations. I taught her about lungs, how to feel for chest expansion, helped her find her heart, taught her to feel for the pulse. Every day, I quizzed her about what was inside as I indicated what was outside, and it became a kind of ritual between us: tell me the name of the thing under this gauze pad I am taping on you, show me where the food goes, show me where it travels inside. Other nurses joined. The direct-care staff, inspired and perhaps emboldened by the novelty of these strange didactic scenes, began stuffing small radios into their pockets and encouraging Sara to dance in her room, narrating body moves as they demonstrated – "this is your right arm shaking up and down," "now we bend to the left," "hands on hips," and so on. Sara began to invent housekeeping chores for herself – wiping the windows and the floor tiles, dusting along the wall edges. Staff allowed her to use towels at first, and then, eventually, a broom from the housekeeper's closet. Together, over a period of months, we built with Sara the metaphorical outlines of an inner landscape, a sense of being embodied, and we enabled her, at the same time, to achieve an intimacy and a mastery of the spaces that were, irreducibly, outside her. We shored up the partitions and made solid the borders eroded by her years of swallowing.

The facility had a particularly compassionate psychologist who started meeting with Sara twice a week. He developed a series of what are called "exposure" exercises, sitting with her in a special therapy room and placing around the table an assortment of objects, starting, in the first weeks, with items too large to fit in her mouth and moving progressively, over time, toward smaller and smaller things. A recreational therapist scheduled time in the gym so that Sara could run around, which we hoped might reduce her need to shove furniture. The gym staff got her a large rubber ball to toss and kick, its outer surfaces quietly repeating, with each touch, the message of separation of me from not me.

Repeated X-rays began to reveal that Sara's swallowing had slowed. She could go for several months without new objects appearing in the abdominal scan. Gradually and in steps, restrictions were lifted: Sara was allowed in an activity room for 30 minutes, first once a day, then twice a day, with one crayon at a time. Then, church services. Then, for 20 minutes at a time, joining the morning and evening unit meetings for coffee in the company of other patients. Then the outdoor porch, with supervision. Eventually, a year and a half after her admission, Sara was able to have a roommate, another patient with a long history of swallowing who had been placed on similar restrictions regarding clothing and personal belongings.

We nurses came to believe we had done some of our best work with Sara – a work of dogged restraint, self-discipline, and almost infinite patience, marked, above all, by a willingness to recognize in her pathology a kind of creativity, something imaginative, albeit grotesque and distorted. Creating physical experiences that gave a form and simple physical representation to a specific idea – reflecting and reinforcing a separation of inside from outside – we had connected to Sara's primary themes, her literal themes of taking in, of making mine, but reconfigured them, setting them, to some extent, on a new course. We "spoke" to Sara – in activities and motions – about borders and boundaries. And though we never fully halted her swallowing, we did, finally, measurably slow it, enabling her to regain a small amount of dignity and independence.

Creative processes in nursing work

What, if anything, was distinctive about the nursing interventions which had worked in this situation to ease Sara's suffering? I decided I would try to pinpoint their specific characteristics. This book, the by-product of my reflections, is about the deployment of metaphoric reasoning in psychiatric and mental health nursing. With examples drawn from the treatment of severely chronically mentally ill patients in a variety of settings, I describe episodes in which psychiatric nursing teams reached past ordinary language and deployed, instead, unconventional methods more akin to art, in key respects, than to traditional nursing practice. Rooted in metaphor, symbol, reference, and analogy, they harnessed the creative and imaginative tools and aesthetic attitude of the artist and the poet rather than the methods more conventionally associated with professional nursing-care planning and understandings of patient care needs. These interventions do not match a box from "column A" to a box from "column B," the nursing action to a preconceived need or objective read-off from a diagnostic list. Rather, they represent a form of aesthetically grounded therapeutic communication which has roots in play therapy with children and is familiar in psychodynamic and psychoanalytic circles but which has not previously been theorized as a part of the nursing toolkit. These methods added significantly to the patients' treatment by opening doors for a therapeutic alliance to begin where previous efforts at engagement had failed.

Psychotherapy privileges the spoken word, and traditional music and art rehabilitation therapies presuppose patients' capacity to cooperate in groups and participate in communicative exchange. None of these can proceed, however, when patients are dangerous, uncooperative, or highly regressed. In the earliest stages of psychiatric hospitalization, with the most severely ill patients whose behaviors make talk-based therapy impractical or impossible, sensitive relationship-building has to come first. At its core, relationship-building is about language. It calls for identifying a specific communicative channel which might enable initial interpersonal contact. In collaborative, multidisciplinary treatment planning of the type which characterizes most inpatient settings, front-line nurses are the personnel to whom this task often falls. We spend far more time observing and interacting with patients than do most other kinds of clinician, which makes it possible for us to achieve a level of intimacy and familiarity, early on, which other clinicians often lack. Moreover, our time tends to be flexible. Not bound by advance scheduling or a need to bill for particular hours of service or sessions of a prescribed length, nurses watch situations unfold in "real time" and can grasp opportunities to build understanding in moments of patients' greatest receptivity.

Some of us might be licensed or trained to conduct manualized therapeutic protocols such as cognitive behavioral therapy or dialectical behavioral therapy, but since most of us are not, our opportunities are wide-ranging for nuanced interventions that emerge directly from patients' observable modes of relating – and, equally importantly, from our own often under-utilized capacity for creative and sensitive engagement in the clinical encounter.

Symptoms, in mental illness, are regarded as signs of disease. But they are also communications. Fragmented, perhaps bizarre, they are pieces of a hieroglyphic-like system which may be decipherable if we take them seriously as salient and meaning-bearing – as windows into the patient's private dialect (Laing, 1969). We nurses are well poised to listen to these symptom dialects, as our profession has been rooted, from the start, in an attunement to the body's speech. We register in our ear canals the poignant whoosh that air makes as it searches the recesses of the collapsing lung. We feel the quickening of our own pulse in tune with the throbbing of a patient's frightened heart. We breathe the saltiness of wounds and find, in those inhalations, surprising moments of mute kinship. Our work trains us in the great diversity of human vocabularies – in the body's plaintive, hesitant whispers, its whines of self-absorption, its joyous declarations and deep-seated groans of anguish – in all its multitude of strange and subtle productions and pronouncements.

All the more so in psychiatric nursing, where our patients' mysterious, sometimes disturbing gestures and psychotic delusions challenge us to reach into the deepest inner dictionaries of connectivity and understanding. To pay attention to these, to be open to meanings embodied even in bizarre presentations, is to call upon Freud's groundbreaking articulation, more than a century ago, of the human capacity for an understanding which is at once generous and intellectually rigorous (Birnbaum, 2015).

Paul Ricoeur, the French philosopher of language who wrote extensively about psychiatric illness and psychotherapy, suggested that to work with the mentally ill, fundamentally, is to reintroduce into the linguistic community those who have been excommunicated from it (Ricoeur, 2012). This book claims for nurses a key role in achieving that re-introduction – deploying a specific kind of technique at a particular moment in the clinical process.

The gestural bridge

How might we describe the nursing interventions deployed in the encounter with Sara? They were empathic and generous, as any nursing interventions should be. But our games and playful activities with her – the call-and-response-style pointing and identifying, the floor-sweeping and surface-wiping, the naming and dancing, and so on – cannot be classified wholly as therapeutic communication in the way nurses generally understand it. There were no uniquely identifiable listening techniques, no set of structured responses, no interactive verbal scripts demonstrating emotional availability, validation, or compassionate presence in the moment. Our intentions were not conveyed by posture, tone, or facial expression. We gave no praise, offered no words of encouragement or reassurance. Nobody talked about their feelings. Nor could our encounters be classified in the same category as talk-based psychotherapy, with its long-range goal of promoting durable insight and conscious self-awareness.

Rather, it can be said that our interactions contained something at once more abstract and more transitional. They harbored a message – embodied in, and delivered through, the structure of the activity itself. Through body-based encounters which configured them gesturally, as a form of analogy, we had found a means to "speak" with Sara about borders and boundaries and about the separation of inside from outside. Giving these ideas an indirect, figurative representation, but without pinning them down in speech, we enabled Sara to constitute her body's boundaries as a mental experience and enabled her to feel them, without having recourse to words or conscious understanding. This is the basis of an approach I call the "gestural bridge."

Gestural bridges are sensory-based play activities which cast psychological ideas in an analogic physical form. They deploy metaphor as a bridge that facilitates initial contact with a patient's private themes before conventional language is available to characterize and convey them. Gestural bridging provides tools that support a patient to order and organize some of the problematic elements which remain private, unnamed, and untamed in his or her felt world – to create a representation for some of his or her internal ideas. Without conventional speech, it builds a shared space of contact and meaning exchange between patient and nurse. Inviting the patient into an indirect kind of conversation – what cognitive linguists have sometimes called a "conceptual metaphor," (Fauconnier & Turner, 2002; Lakoff & Johnson, 1999) – it creates conditions for movement forward into treatment alliance.

It is the goal of this book to describe the gestural bridge in a way that makes it accessible and understandable for mental health clinicians, particularly nurses, who work with very challenging and persistently ill patients who have not responded to conventional treatment approaches. In subsequent chapters, I discuss the philosophical and developmental underpinnings of this technique and illustrate its use with examples drawn from a variety of care settings.

Organization of the book

Various details in these stories have been altered. This preserves anonymity and confidentiality for people and organizations. But while the descriptions here cannot be said to represent any specific clinical facility or program, readers in the mental health field will recognize easily the policies, procedures, and presentations common to most, if not all, contemporary psychiatric and mental health settings where people register for treatment when they are very severely ill. Each of the examples here illustrates a situation in which a patient presented what we commonly call "a problem" – a persistent lack of response to conventional treatments. In each situation, the patient remained behaviorally disorganized, even after weeks or months of effort by clinical teams. "Gestural bridge" activities are described which, in each situation, enabled personal themes to be explored and expressed in a way that effected a kind of clinical pivot for the patient – enabling a transition toward engagement in treatment and more conventional language and behavior. Chapter 3 reviews some of the logical and philosophical underpinnings of this approach, linking gestural bridging to work in the history of more established methods for deploying play and metaphor in the therapeutic encounter. Additional examples are then followed, in Chapter 7, by a discussion of implications for nursing education and professional preparation.

The pages which follow contain no narratives of redemption. Patients did not get well in a magic-wand moment; nor did they get well quickly. Since few studies track long-term life outcomes for patients in psychiatric care, it isn't even possible to claim durability for the results. Rather, the interventions described here were relatively short-term measures of desperation, lasting on the order of weeks or days, aimed at reaching patients who had not responded to other forms of invitation to a treatment alliance. These interventions served not as the whole of treatment – far from it – but rather as a transitional phase, an opening gate through which more intensive and longer-lasting clinical work could be launched, mostly by clinicians outside of nursing. The stories here highlight contributions which nurses are poised to make at specific and mostly early points in the interdisciplinary clinical process as a result of our uniquely intimate access to patients – so long as we are willing to expand our understanding of what it means to communicate therapeutically. They illustrate the "gestural bridge" as a creative therapeutic art that can emerge in the context of nurses' intensely personal and intimate contact with patients.

I am a nurse and educator and have been an artist for many years, and this combination generates a perspective which inevitably informs and affects my work. But a wide variety of clinicians – social workers, psychologists, music and art therapists, and addictions counselors, for example – will find their struggles and experiences reflected here, as the core aims of connection and authentic communication are shared throughout the mental health and human development professions. More academically minded readers will discover here some practical applications of recent theoretical work in such areas as cognitive linguistics, metaphor studies, and the philosophy of art and consciousness, subjects which will be touched on briefly later in the book.

Note

1 Portions of this chapter have appeared previously in Birnbaum, S. (2015). Freud still matters to nursing: a response to Sandra P. Thomas. *Issues in Mental Health Nursing* 36, 1017–1018. Reprinted by permission of Taylor & Francis.

References

Birnbaum, S. (2015). Freud still matters to nursing: a response to Sandra P. Thomas. *Issues in Mental Health Nursing* 36, 1017–1018.

Fauconnier, G. & Turner, M. (2002). *The way we think: Conceptual blending and mind's hidden complexities.* New York, NY: Basic Books.

Laing, R.D. (1969). *The divided self.* New York, NY: Penguin Books.

Lakoff, G. & Johnson, M. (1999). *Philosophy in the flesh: The embodied mind and its challenge to western thought.* New York, NY: Basic Books.

Ricoeur, P. (2012). *The rule of metaphor: Multidisciplinary studies of the creation of meaning in language.* Toronto, Ont.: University of Toronto Press.

2 The gestural bridge

Joe had attended college briefly and worked part-time as a disc jockey for a local radio station. Fired from the job after repeated sobbing outbursts, he ran out of money and became homeless following eviction from a rental apartment. Police found him wandering along the side of a road. Hospitalized for psychiatric care, he was started on medications and then released. Unable to access supports from among locally available community service options, however, he rapidly decompensated and was soon returned for inpatient care following a series of suicide attempts by drug overdose. In the new setting, Joe confined himself to a corner chair near a window in the day room. When he wasn't slumped under a winter coat as the TV blared, he wandered the small hallway, tearful or, sometimes, in full-throttle sobbing. Multiple medication trials did not break this odd cast, even after many weeks. Disappointment and despair set in among the clinical staff.

If anyone attempted to strike up conversation, Joe would launch into a bizarre fusillade of sobbing complaints: I can't read, I can't think, I can't see straight, he would insist tearfully. My legs hurt, my arms feel heavy, I can't remember things, I can't listen to music, I don't enjoy anything. Staff and patients alike found these punishing tirades disturbing and began to avoid Joe, as nobody wanted to set off another barrage. The facility had recently seen a suicide attempt; the attending psychiatrist, wary about copy-catting, placed Joe on close-monitoring status, specifying that he spend some time each day talking privately with a nurse as yet another round of new trial medications was started.

They teach you in nursing school to "establish rapport," and that, very simply, was the starting objective for the nursing team. I invited Joe to join me in one of the activity rooms. But every day for a week, our meetings were chaotic and unpleasant, as Joe sank deeply into any available chair, teary-eyed, and sooner or later began torturing his arms and thighs with alarmingly compulsive scraping gestures of his fingernails. Between sobs, he fired off the familiar I-can't-see-I-can't-think-I-can't-focus, and so on. Though I documented faithfully my nursing intervention – "supportive counseling and empathic listening" – I didn't feel my "counseling" was particularly supportive, and my listening didn't feel the least bit "empathic." I certainly could see why the staff found Joe so difficult to tolerate.

The facility had a sunny backyard. Perhaps a little fresh air and sunshine, I thought, might help this guy. So, one day, I took our sessions outdoors. The heaving sobs, the fingernail scraping, the litany of this and that gone wrong – it all came predictably as Joe slumped his shoulders and sank into the park bench.

Presence alone, as we're taught in nursing school, has the capacity to soothe and console. "Therapeutic use of self," I reminded myself. But outdoors, as indoors, I felt again the uniquely unpleasant sensation of being compressed, inundated, by Joe's aggressive brand of misery and incessant harping. You're not supposed to look away from your patient – that's Nursing Communication 101 – but I found myself gazing guiltily at the quiet, tree-covered hill beyond the fence, my eyes seeking relief in a more open vista.

People caution you not to "take your work home." But one night, a strange memory came to me of an episode, years earlier, when a small bat had flown into the window of my ninth-floor New York City apartment. Panicked and desperate, it frantically slammed itself against walls and knocked pictures off their hooks. Several of us had exhausted ourselves in the effort to trap and free it. I thought now about the frenetic tone of someone who is exhausting himself – and everyone around him – trying to locate himself in an open, unfamiliar space. My mind traveled, too, to the story from classical mythology of Pan, the Greek god, who has the body of a man and the head and legs of a goat. Pan is so ugly that everyone retreats from him. One day, he comes across a nymph named Syrinx. Falling instantly in love, he chases her, but she runs away, seeking refuge in a river, where her sisters hide her by transforming her into a reed. As the wind blows, a melody is produced. Pan stands, mesmerized. Not knowing which reed is Syrinx, he grabs a handful and ties them quickly together side by side. Forever after, their music in the wind – the music of Pan's pipe – evokes for him the presence of his lost love. Our word for "syringe" is derived from this story, as is our word for "panic." More importantly, as the philosopher Ernst Bloch once noted, the ancient story speaks to our fundamental understanding of sound's remarkable capacity to evoke form, or, as Bloch states poetically, "to trace, in the invisible, the outlines of human longing" (Bloch, 1985, p. 197). Which brings us to the nursing intervention that suddenly registered itself in my mind.

Most of us, at an early age, learn to soothe ourselves when we feel lost. We linger in hot showers and wrap ourselves in plush towels. We snuggle under blankets, embrace furry pets, and slather on floral-scented lotions which envelope our bodies in comforting, familiar associations. We conjure shapes and surfaces of texture and temperature and scent which remind us about companionship and enclosure. Joe's gestural patterns – the sinking deeply into chairs, the wrapping under absurdly seasonally inappropriate winter coats, the scratching to heighten sensations at the body surface – all these, I realized, could be read as a kind of frantic effort to evoke for himself a feeling of enclosure, of boundedness in space. The more I reflected on it, the more it seemed we were all feeling cramped around Joe because something about his lurching tirades and constant tearfulness amounted, essentially, to an aggressive projection of force against surfaces.

Anyone who has cradled children in lullabies or attended choir services in large cathedrals knows viscerally the unique feel that sound exerts on the body's membranes. Sound by itself, as the Pan story reminds us, has the capacity to create form and texture – to manipulate air into shapes that soothe and surround with minutely felt gradations of pressure and motion. Joe had worked in radio: he'd come to us from the world of sound. It made sense, now, to consider that sound itself might form the basis of a more productive means of making contact with him.

Next time we sat outside, I asked Joe if he'd ever incorporated nature or animal sounds in any of the radio shows he had done before his hospitalizations. He remembered using whale recordings, and I told him that I wanted him to think, now, about those old recordings, and to try listening to the sounds outside us. I scooted alongside him, and we turned our faces outward together.

At first, we heard the rumbling of an airplane engine overhead. Then, we heard the heaving groans of the facility electrical-power generators. We heard the crackle of truck wheels scraping gravel at a construction site down the road. We heard the whine of flies, the Morse code of woodpeckers, the hurrying trill of wrens and fleetingly, beyond that, the distant bustle of traffic. The cosmos cooperated with this experiment, thankfully, offering rich sequences of varied and nuanced noises. Given the specific assignment of listening, it was clear, Joe could still himself, at least for a short period, as my sitting alongside him served as a wordless initiation of collaboration and synchrony.

The following day, we tried again. I began pointing to each sound as we heard it. This time, I asked Joe not just to listen, but to try envisioning the location of each sound and to imagine, much the way a blind man uses a cane, the three-dimensional physical space between the sound points – to translate, in a sense, from the auditory to the visual and tactile experience of geographical space. For a week of these brief interventions, lasting no more than 10 or 15 minutes each time, we played this "blind-man" game. We mentally constructed all manner of spaces – cubes and domes and so on – from cricket chatter, ambulance sirens, bird calls and whatever else was available. Step by step, in this way, I re-acquainted Joe with his capacity to hear, and, indirectly, to sense in other ways – to see and feel the spaces around him. And in a more general sense to deploy the mind's eye and remember what might, constructively, be done with it. Joe continued to cry silently.

By the second week of this activity, however, I noticed that the subject matter of Joe's speech started gradually to broaden. He began speculating about measurable distances such as the number of yards to the nearest highway and the square footage between bird calls. He lowered the volume of his voice. The crying diminished. He began telling me about playing the guitar (both of us had taken lessons), about his family, about apartments he'd lived in or visited over the years. The themes made sense: sound, space, the familiar surfaces of people and place – all following along a widening trail of ideas set out by the activity of our listening, seeing, and imagining together. By the third week, the sobbing stopped. The complaining stopped.

I continued to document the nursing intervention: "supportive counseling and empathic listening." But these phrases described inadequately the inchoate but palpable shift I had observed. In the vocabulary of sound – in the delicate mutuality of our seeking it, without my using words to pin him down or trap him in conversations he wasn't ready to have – Joe seemed to be grasping a sense not only of *location*, but of *being located*. Of possessing within himself a capacity to narrate a personal envelope.

On the ward floor, staff noted that Joe started waking for breakfast and joining the staff-and-patient morning group meeting. He attended first one and then more of his assigned group programs. The scratching gestures had ceased. Removed from close monitoring, Joe was able to begin earning points toward a less restrictive level of supervision – to gain more independence and grounds privileges. Soon, he began attending regularly scheduled sessions with his doctors and therapists; he enrolled in music classes. Everyone on the staff felt that medications had worked, programming had worked, nursing had worked. He even made a few friends. As his schedule filled, he and I stopped our regular meetings. There was no longer a need for them. His therapist told me a few weeks later that he was looking for an apartment, preparing for re-entry into community life, and, more importantly, eager to reconnect with family, friends, and work, feeling optimistic for his future prospects.

Making contact when words are not available

It is not difficult to notice that the stories of Sara and Joe share a common thread, despite their outward differences. Each begins with a patient who is isolated and suffering, unable or unwilling, for one reason or another, to enter productively into conventional therapeutic programs or treatments, who is alienated from the day-to-day world of ordinary human conversation. Then, something happens between patient and nurse. An interaction changes things. It begins with the nurse's alertness to a pattern, gesture, or other element of behavior which is specific and unique to the patient, but which lends itself to reconstruction in the form of a simple, time-limited game or activity. The game or activity is direct and straightforward – easily grasped. It requires no jargon-laden theoretical elaboration, no translation, no complicated manual of step-by-step instructions. It is playful and accessible. Anyone can do it. It incorporates many of the traditional therapeutic competencies – the show of attention, of empathy, of patience and confidence and compassion, the sense of genuineness and emotional availability, the commitment to establishing a protective interpersonal sanctuary, a holding environment, which is nourishing and stable. But the activity's most important feature is precisely something else: it embodies a specific logical subject matter distinct from these other attributes. It gives body-based physical form to a specific but abstract idea. It creates a *representability* for something the patient has been unable previously to name – something which now can be shared, in the form of a conceptual analogy, in the play between patient and nurse.

Vocabulary shift

In the encounter with Joe, as in the encounter with Sara, we can identify a specific logical transformation. Emerging from Joe's distinctive relationship with music and sound, a "blind man's" listening game became an alternative, viscerally based vocabulary for suggesting to him, without words, the themes of safety, mutuality, and the possibility of invoking the feeling of a safe, enveloping surface of personal space – something akin to what psychoanalyst Didier Anzieu called "the skin ego" (Anzieu, 2016). Starting with his appreciation for music and sound – with his personal idiom rather than with more conventional therapeutic language – the game invited him into an activity which expressed, to some extent, what was plaguing him, but in an alternate, sensory vocabulary that was accessible, familiar, and non-threatening. Over his aggressive and disturbing emotional flailing, his grasping for boundaries and containment, the game cast a new, plainer structure, the suggestion of a more orderly and coherent representation.

We attain what is possible, it is sometimes said, by extending what is given; we employ the known to invent what has not been known previously. The activities described here embody this common-sense principle. Starting with elements of the patient's own communicative system, but recasting them in an accessible, body-based vocabulary which can be shared and elaborated by someone else we were able to initiate our patients into an exchange of meanings, around themes of keen interest, but without rushing them into conversations they were not ready to have or group programs they were not ready to endure. This transformation is what I am calling the "gestural bridge." The capacity for therapeutic communication of this type has not previously been theorized in nursing. But it has been the subject of considerable attention in other disciplines, particularly cognitive linguistics, philosophy, art, and psychoanalysis, and it has roots, as will be seen, in the earliest communicative encounters of infants and children. This is the subject of the next chapter.

References

Anzieu, D. (2016). *The skin-ego* (N. Segal, Trans.). London: Karnac.

Bloch, E. (1985). *Essays on the philosophy of music*. New York, NY: Cambridge University Press.

3 Metaphor, play, and the representation of ideas in body-based analogy: meeting people where they are

What happens, actually, in the encounter between patient and psychiatric nurse? What makes this kind of contact feel special? More importantly, what makes it useful to patients? Even our richest theorizing tends to turn vague at precisely the moment of the encounter itself. References to "intersubjectivity," "unknowability," "relationality" and shared meanings, and so on, are commonplace in our professional literature, especially at the advanced level, and they speak to something that feels true – to a feeling of connection and solidarity, of genuine mutuality, which all of us know well. But they do little to describe the specific logical structure of the transformations that unfold in the actual context of an interpersonal exchange. They might even, to some extent, be misleading, or, perhaps worse, presumptuous, since no one, after all, can really claim unequivocally to have visited the inside of another mind. So let us examine the interactions described here and identify their logical content and structure and the nature of what they accomplished for the patients.

The nursing interventions with Sara and Joe both appeared, initially, as ordinary play. They were games. The patients participated naturally, without anything seeming forced or contrived. No words of praise or encouragement had to be offered. No special training or preparation was required. But the games had a distinctive mental impact. Without conventional therapeutic language, they established the incipient possibility of communicability around an issue which previously had remained beyond the patient's reach of speaking and naming. It might be said that a kind of translation was effected. It started with a private, isolating kind of experiencing, and it turned into something more externally representable and share-able with others – though not quite ready to be characterized in words. To understand this approach and how it works, how it unlocks the possibility of therapeutic contact, we can examine key features of its structure and form. In this chapter, we will look first at what is ordinary and play-like about the gestural bridge and second at what is evocative and powerful in its distinctive logical configuration.

The dual structure of play

Let us consider, first, the structure of ordinary play. If you've played a game with anyone, you know this: in order to play, you've got to submit to a system of shared, concrete rules. Think of basketball, tennis, chess, hide-and-seek. Each requires some measure of acquiescence – to turn-taking, to timing, to court-boundary lines and equipment and technique, and so on. These are the limitations in the game which every player needs to know and which define each game as a unique and distinct activity – as this particular game and not another. Limits give a game its familiarity and stability – its know-ability and share-ability.

At the same time, however, what gives pleasure and satisfaction in a game is what does not relate to its limits and rules: the moves nobody predicts in advance, the surprises which the players reveal as they play. These give a game its vitality and its spontaneity – they make it worth our while to join and to observe. You might play a game a million times, but in every episode of play, the irreducible polarity is re-created: the constraints of the familiar, of the shared rules, are met by the potential, equally strong, for the arrival of something new, something which is exerted by the will of each player as an individual, in the specific context of the unfolding moment. This is true not just for games played jointly, but, in certain respects, for solitary play as well. Consider, for example, the child leaping from the boulder. She accepts, perhaps grudgingly, the limitations imposed by gravity. But each time she jumps, she discovers how much higher or farther it might be possible to go.

The same can be said about art, which we might regard as a serious variety of play. Between the painter and the canvas, between the composer and the musical instrument, between the poet and his language, fundamental limitations exist – the flatness of the fabric on the frame, for example, the vocabularies and cadences given by dialect and tradition, the sound-frequency range of even the best-made instrument, and so on. The artist concedes to these objective limits in his or her choice of medium. But even so, the canvas cannot predict the painting, nor the instrument predict the melody, just as the boulder cannot predict the leap, and the rules of a game cannot determine in advance the sportsmanship and athleticism which might be displayed by its players. We might say, more simply, that a conversation unfolds, in the structure of play, between what is bounded and what is unbounded, between what is contained and what might be released.

This duality is inscribed early in the human experience of play, and researchers believe it is implicated at the core of our capacity for making and sharing meaning with others (Akhtar, 2011; Ammaniti & Stern, 1994; Bruner, Jolly, & Sylva, 1976). Long before an infant understands what language is, his parent (or other caregiver) engages him in a kind of play. She hugs and cradles him, returns his smiles, laughs at his cooing, reflects back his curious gazes. She extends her arms to swing him joyously airborne, and she reclaims him, giggling, to her close embrace. Over time, in the course of these affectionate exchanges, a system of meanings coalesces; *significance* takes form around mutually comprehensible gestures and motions. The infant develops, with the parent, a kind of action language – a body-based dialogue which assigns predictable gestural configurations to feelings and intentions. The infant learns to initiate communications in ways which elicit response, and so, in turn, does the parent. An enormously significant personal and cognitive transformation unfolds here – with an impact which is both mental and emotional: conceptual discretion is born in the infant. The infant learns what it means to be able to *acknowledge* – to impose intentional frames of identification around still-inchoate elements of experience. He or she is introduced, in other words, to the possibility of *representation* – to the capacity for wresting the tell-able, the identifiable, from what previously, just days or weeks or months earlier, did not exist as a category. Moreover, the back-and-forth motion of this parent–child play, its alternating hesitations and revelations, its opportunities for delay and surprise, inscribes in the infant a bodily grasp of what it means to predict and expect, to disclose and discover, to concede and withhold, and so on. Child and parent build a "language" between them that bridges what is private and internal with what potentially can be called up for sharing externally.

So crucial and formative for the child is this early period of creating playfully, with another person, a system of meanings incorporating both private and shared elements, the celebrated British psychoanalyst Donald Winnicott (Winnicott, 2010) among others, regarded it as the very birthplace of psychological well-being. It marks the inception, Winnicott believed, of the child's sense of having capacity and personal agency *vis-à-vis* other people and the world. The gestural bridging approach described here emerges from this early capacity for deliberate creation, between people, of meaning-bearing dialects which are not dependent on conventional spoken language. It draws from the fundamental duality in the structure of playful exchange – from its straddling of open-endedness and rule-boundedness, its capacity to ground a person in what is externally share-able while linking, at the same time, to personally held associations, meanings, and individual potentialities.

The nature of metaphor

As we might remember from secondary school, metaphor is the name given to a statement with the implicit or explicit structure "A-is-B." It is an instance of something being represented indirectly, analogically, in terms of something else. The word "metaphor" comes to us from the ancient Greek word *metapherein*, which means "to transport" or "to carry," and metaphors have long been a subject of interest to scholars because of their unique power "to carry" ideas in literature and art. Dating as far back as the time of Aristotle, in fact, countless philosophers, theologians, artists, linguists, literary theorists, and, more recently, cognitive scientists have studied extensively the logical structure of the process which unfolds when we use a metaphor in writing or speech. Theorists propose that metaphors convey something which is simultaneously the same as, and also different from, our private experience (Gerhart & Russell, 1984; Gibbs, 1994; Gibbs & Colston, 2012; Johnson, 1987, 2007; Lakoff & Johnson, 1980; Lakoff & Turner, 1989; Radman, 1997). They harbor something near and also something far, initiating a dialogue between old and new. A word or phrase may have familiar qualities which refer or connect, perhaps uncannily, to what is immediate and personal in the life of the listener or reader. But a vagueness and indeterminacy in that same word or phrase may call up, at the same time, new associations which were not present before, in new domains of thought and feeling. Metaphor, in other words, shares with play its characteristic duality of form. It straddles openness and closure.

Many of us might remember the chilling poem "The Waste Land," a classic of modern literature. T.S. Eliot's most famous work, it cited widely, offers a useful illustration about the structure of metaphors and the way they "work" in our minds. Consider the line:

> A woman drew her long black hair out tight,
> And fiddled whispered music on those strings.
> (Eliot, 2001, p. 18)

The first part of this statement, we can see, is literal and concrete. It describes the visual image of a woman brushing her hair. But the second part is metaphorical: connecting hair with strings, brushing with fiddling and whispering, it transports our associations from a simple concrete image to visual, auditory, and other physical and emotional domains of experience. It conjures violinists, melodies, the delicate touch of bow on string, the internal modulation and fine-muscular restraint we muster in the act of whispering, the aching suggestiveness of something whispered, the pain of hair being pulled, the act of talking to ourselves with an internal whispered voice, and the often eerie, sometimes foreboding way in which sound registers in parts of our bodies other than the ears and mouth. And so on. The lines might strike different chords in each person who reads them. But common to all is the sense of finding oneself unlocked from purely specific meanings as the metaphor configures a bridge between the here-and-now and the something-else, somewhere-else, the some-other-time and some-other-sense. The metaphor's power, as literary critic Denis Donoghue has written (Donoghue, 2014), is in the capacity to conjure through an array of allusions, references, and implications – to create new thought connections from old ones.

Metaphors have a characteristic directionality, scholars have observed: When we deploy them to understand one concept in terms of another, we tend to structure the vaguer and more elusive concepts – like those for emotions, spiritual awareness, or aesthetic experiences – in terms which are more concretely understood in direct, body-based, physical ways. Think of how understandable we become, for example, when we say that a relationship is "on a rocky road" or "going downhill," that a situation at work is "thorny" or "sticky," that someone is "cold" or his personality "magnetic," that "an idea slipped my mind" or that we were "wounded by a cutting remark." Theorists refer to directionality of this type as a "conceptual mapping" of complex, abstract ideas on to more concrete bodily "source" knowledge (Gibbs, 1994, 2008) and have noted the remarkable vividness, clarity, and richness of information which "mappings" of this type facilitate in communicative exchange (Johnson, 1987).

References to size, shape, height, depth, weight, temperature, direction, and other fundamental physical and sense-based properties figure especially prominently when we deploy metaphoric mappings to relay emotional ideas or describe the intensity with which we feel them. When a person is kind, for example, we say he is "warmhearted." When he is generous, "big-hearted." When he's had trouble in love, "broken-hearted." If he is regretful, "heavy-hearted." Both in our minds and in our bodies, it is easy to feel what is meant by phrases like "burning shame," "bitter disappointment," or "cold shoulder." We know what it means to "get an impression" – as if sensibility itself were made of clay.

Cross-sensory correspondences: conversations without words

Underlying metaphoric mappings is meaning's strange capacity to wander in the body, as ideas speak to one another across the domains of lived experience. Scientists refer to this phenomenon as "cross-modality," or "the unity of the senses" (Stern, 1985), and have observed its centrality in child development. At the start of an infant's life, neuropsychologist Daniel Stern has noted, infants and parents register and exchange information with one another through a rich (and delightful) variety of sounds, gestures, and facial expressions which signal intensity, shape, size, quantity, and so on. Subjective states such as exuberance, for example, may be expressed vocally (the gleeful squeal), gesturally (the wiggly dance or joyous outstretching of arms), or as facial display (the beaming smile), and perhaps in other ways as well. Their intensity may be amplified or modulated through tone and volume, degrees of muscular flexion and extension, pace and direction, rhythm and repetition, and so on. Each expressive form confers its own unique features, and yet all of them, even without words, are completely recognizable (Stern, 1985).

Without our conscious awareness of it, cross-modality informs a great many of our everyday judgments and assessments. Consider, for example, how the corner florist's carefully arranged bouquets can evoke so remarkably the optimism of a wedding, the solemnity of a funeral, or the ache and depth of a lover's yearning. Or how the paint-maker's color mixtures call up with such clarity and precision the celebratory, festive, or calming mood you were hoping to invoke in your dining room or bath renovation. How many of us, following a satisfying restaurant meal, have described a particularly pleasing side dish or dessert in terms like "vibrant" or "robust" – metaphoric words which are not at all related to flavor but are completely appropriate and comprehensible nonetheless? Think of the winemaker and the perfumer, who arouse by allusion through the medium of scent, or the dressmaker, whose choice of lush fabrics speaks volumes about physical desire. "The flash of thought and its swiftness explain the lightning flash," Helen Keller famously observed about the multiplicity and multidirectionality of cross-modal metaphoric connections which enabled her to reach across the gulf of deafness and blindness to grasp the world outside herself. "I recognize truth by the clearness and guidance it gives my thought... Knowing what that clearness is, I can imagine what light is to the eye" (Keller, 2009, p. 53).

Connections such as these – which philosopher Susanne Langer called "congruences of form" (Langer, 1953, p. 27) – are a key to the power of symbolic expression throughout the arts, accounting, in part, for the capacity of art to "move" and "impress" (words which are themselves metaphorical) across gulfs of culture and time, regardless of any specific medium. Think of the color splashes that pulse across a painting: traversing vision, motion, and sound as they call up the sense of a pounding headache or a heart throbbing inside a chest. Or the repetition of words such as "here" or "now" in parts of a poem, insinuating, as we read aloud, the recurring emotional tug, the insistence of people and stories remembered, the sensation of which a mathematician might cast in the form of a sine wave. More than one music theorist has observed the ways tone amplitude suggests amplitude of movement, and variations in the duration and length of silences or musical notes can suggest kinetic contours such as the spiral, the descent, and the swirl (Margulis, 2014; Nattiez, 1998; Patel, 2008) – themselves motions which are rich in personal references and therefore moving or meaningful to us when we see them, for example, in ballet or modern dance. "Music," wrote Langer, "is the tonal analogue of emotional life" (Langer, 1953, p. 27). Along these lines, it is not hard to call to mind the unique musical note that announces a favored song's refrain, telling the ear where an idea begins and then, perhaps maddeningly, begins again – the return of something which will not allow itself to be ignored.

We've all met people who "talk with their hands." Linguists have coined the term "metaphorics" for the familiar but unconscious body gestures that accompany speech and convey meanings, often without the need for words (McNeil, 1987, 1992). Many of us use our arms, for example, to indicate "this big" when telling how much we love someone. We squeeze our fists together urgently, prayer-like, when we describe intense desire – as if ready to grasp it tight, right in the moment, and not let it go. Think of how commonplace it is to hold out a hand in a palm-upward position when saying "may I ask you a question?" – as if the hand, like a cup, might be ready to receive the stuff of an answer. Metaphorically rich gestures and motions such as these are well known in education: who among us can't remember the math teacher gesturing frantically upward, downward, or across his or her own body when explaining equations and logarithmic functions that "approach" zero, "tend" toward infinity, or "pass through" an axis (Lakoff & Nunez, 2000)? Many of us can call to mind quite clearly – and perhaps fondly – the writing teacher who gestured "explosions" with her hands, admonishing us to make our ideas "pop" on the written page.

Educational psychologists and other scholars in recent years have demonstrated that in a great variety of contexts where one person is striving to shape the understanding of another, metaphoric cross-modalities often play a central role. Teachers change vocal tones, move hands or arms, shift body positions, and so on, showing one thing in terms of another as they encourage students to map abstract concepts on to more concrete and accessible bodily schemas. Bodily gestures and postures are many teachers' way of using familiar stories and domains of experience to guide learners toward using their own experience to create new conceptual mappings and reason in new ways (Cienki & Muller, 2008; Fauconnier & Turner, 2002; Turner, 1996; Williams, 2008).

In all of these commonplace analogies, at home and in school as in literature and the fine arts, our metaphoric mappings are profoundly aesthetically "charged" – they speak to us across a circuit of references and allusions, connecting feeling to representation through links of body experience (Johnson, 2007). They traffic in what psychoanalyst Arnold Modell has called "the currency of the emotional mind" (Modell, 2003). Most importantly, for our purposes in the therapeutic context, they enable concepts and meanings to be exchanged by a great variety of means beyond the spoken word.

Metaphor in mental health work

Let us step back for a moment and consider the many ways metaphor has been understood and deployed previously in mental health work. Theorists and practitioners representing a variety of conceptual approaches and diverse schools of thought have all noted that emotional allusions are often deeply embedded in metaphorical statements, and that symbolic and figurative references serve as clues to unconscious systems of meaning. Think of phrases such as "he barges in like a locomotive," "I feel I hit a wall," or "I was crushed by that remark" – statements familiar in the therapeutic context. To consider these carefully is to come closer to understanding the nuances of what a patient might be thinking and feeling (Combs & Freeman, 1990; Kopp, 1995; McMullen, 2008; Pollio, Barlow, Fine, & Pollio, 1977). Throughout nursing and medicine, researchers have shown that illness and recovery narratives tend to be highly figurative and metaphoric – that patients use a great variety of somatic and environmental references and analogies to make sense of their situations and explain them to others (Charon, 2006; Thomas & Pollio, 2002). Scholars have suggested that metaphors derive their value from their position in between rational, logical, conscious thinking (what psychologists call secondary process) and the more irrational, illogical, collage-like kind of thinking – rich in visual images and lacking sense of time or causal sequence – that dominates in dreams (what psychologists call primary process) (Siegelman, 1990). Tapping into these makes it possible to turn a patient's own language into a focal point for reflection and elaboration and enables clinical workers to introduce or explore ideas indirectly which might be too painful, complicated, or embarrassing to be addressed in more direct ways.

Metaphoric reasoning has figured centrally in the history of psycho-analytic approaches to treatment. More than a century ago, Sigmund Freud struggled to treat emotionally anguished patients suffering inexplicable physical symptoms – a broken-hearted woman experiencing literally, for example, the feeling of being stabbed in the chest. These encounters led him to invent a theory infused throughout with metaphors. Freud conceived of dreams, for example, as a "factory for thought" and a "royal road" to the unconscious and attempted to name specific logical transformations – condensation, displacement, secondary revision, and so on – by which meanings twist metaphorically into symptoms and dream content (Freud, 1955). At the time Freud worked, important new theories were emerging depicting speech and language functions as a series of reflex arcs based in anatomical structures – the "speech centers" of the brain. Freud cautioned, however, that language is too multilayered and complex to be anatomically localized. Memories, intentions, emotions, and physical sensations, he theorized, must be interconnected to language and to each other somehow through a broader and more complex, widely spread system of "associations" for which no scientific explanation had yet been uncovered (Freud, 1953).

What is remarkable, as Ana-Maria Rizzuto has noted in her writings on this issue (Rizzuto, 2013), is the degree to which Freud anticipated current-day neuroscientific and cognitive-science research into what is sometimes now called "the biology of meaning" (Edelman & Tononi, 2000). This is an emerging and expanding interdisciplinary science which seeks to "bring the body back into the mind" (Johnson, 1987) – identifying cellular, chemical, and neurophysiological processes taking place during communication and meaning exchange. New lines of research into such areas as "embodied simulation," "mirror neurons," "neural networks," and "neural enactment" (Ammaniti & Gallese, 2014; Coulson, 2008; Gibbs & Colston, 2012; Varela, Thompson, & Rosch, 1991), and so on, are creating, perhaps not surprisingly, a revival of interest in dynamic psychotherapeutic approaches where metaphorical reasoning and aesthetic judgment are considered central to clinical work (Arieti, 1976; Bollas, 2009; Bollas & Jemstedt, 2011; Borbely, 2008, 2013; Botella & Botella, 2005, 2013; Civitarese, 2013; Katz, 2013; Modell, 2003, 2013; Rothenberg, 1988, 2014).

Explicit use of play activities in therapy dates back to the early period of psychoanalysis, when Melanie Klein and Anna Freud first began using toys in the treatment of child patients. Play was seen as a substitute for the verbal free association which formed the core of adult psychoanalytic treatment. At a time in a person's life when vocabulary is not well developed, these theorists observed, play becomes a language by which children can narrate their experience and give form to their ideas, constituting categories of thought and feeling around which words have not yet coalesced (Marans, Mays, & Colonna, 1993; Solnit, Cohen, & Neubauer, 1993). Rudolf Eckstein, who worked with severely disturbed children in California in the 1960s, described ways of entering into patients' worlds by using their own language and images, harnessing the distinctive communicative idiom which the children themselves were bringing to the therapeutic encounter (Eckstein, 1966). Theorists from a variety of schools of thought have noted that, for adults as well for children, narrative-making can unfold in auditory, kinesthetic, and visual modalities as well as in spoken exchange, and that any of these can be facilitated in the therapeutic context (Axline, 1969, 1974; Freeman, Epston, & Lobovits, 1997; Landreth, 2012; O'Connor, Schaefer, & Braverman, 2015). Dance and "movement" therapists in particular have been at the forefront of research into the ways body-based activity enables metaphoric exploration of trauma and other mental health concerns (Koch, Fuchs, Summa, & Muller, 2012).

Which brings us to the clinical challenge addressed here: what happens when patients lack capacity for conventional communication through language? How do we initiate contact with people who are violent, aggressive, highly regressed, withdrawn, or profoundly bizarre – who are unwilling or unable to tolerate or participate in spoken-word therapies, individually or in groups, and who lack even basic conventional vocabulary for receiving or conveying nuances of thought and feeling? At the earliest stages of treatment, for patients such as these, we need to start somewhere else. We identify an alternate approach that enables us to meet them where they are. This is the function of the gestural bridge.

Play and representation in the gestural bridge

Gestural bridging is an example of what psycholinguists call "conceptual metaphor" (Cienki & Muller, 2008; Fauconnier & Turner, 2002; Lakoff & Johnson, 1980). It begins with the body – the "source" of the cross-modal metaphorical mappings identified by cognitive-science theorists. It begins with a patient's observable behavior or uniquely personal pattern of interaction. An activity or game is developed. The activity touches on core qualities of an idea, core themes of interest to the patient. In an accessible, body-based language, it speaks to something private and idiosyncratic. But it suggests, at the same time, ideas and images brought in from the outside. The structure of the activity enables a connection between something interior in the patient and something which is external and can be held in common with others. Like handing over a basketball and waiting to see what the other player might do with it, it provides the patient with a tool he knows, while challenging him to call up new personal resources. By power of plain suggestion, it activates previously untapped sensibilities and brings them, so to speak, into the playing field.

Like play encounters between a parent and a child, gestural bridges initiate a non-verbal communicative structure which enables the patient to represent ideas outside himself. No one is forced into having conversations he does not want to have. No one is required to name his feelings, identify his personal problems, or acknowledge in any overt way that the nurse has surmised anything about what is troubling him. Instead, a metaphor, deployed playfully, works by the force of its own logic – by the structural fact of its quietly containing an idea that straddles private references and shared ones. This is what connects gestural bridging to metaphoric processes in art and play and distinguishes it from more instrumental and directive approaches in conventional nursing and therapeutic communication.

Gestural interventions as nursing communication

"A new word," wrote the philosopher Ludwig Wittgenstein in 1929, "is like a fresh seed sown on the ground of the discussion" (Wittgenstein, 1980, p. 2). So, too, for what the nurse introduces by means of a gestural bridge. Our "blind man's game" introduced to Joe the suggestion that sounds and physical spaces might be connected to one another. It insinuated that building materials in one sensory modality might be analogous to building materials in another, and by extension, that internal emotional configurations might be analogous to what is perceivable in the outside world. We could not predict what Joe might do with this quietly embedded metaphorical suggestion. But we could see that his thinking was affected in the taking up of the game. Something changed in his mental experience which broke the cast of his previous suffering.

So, too, for the activities we developed with Sara. Our activities directed her attention to boundaries and edges, to the physical distinctness of outsides and insides. They suggested, implicitly, an analogy between external physical boundaries and internal ones. We couldn't see into her mind to understand where she took this mental concept. And she herself lacked the ability to name and discuss it directly. But we could observe, on the surface, the evidence of a strengthened capacity to refrain from violating her body's own internal borders. The theorist Erik

Erikson regarded play as an "emotional laboratory" for the growth of thought (Erikson, 1950, 1968) – a way station where developing minds try out new concepts and representations, acting ideas and experiencing them mentally before being able to speak them or frame them in words. This is the core of the gestural bridge.

"Forms of representation both reveal and conceal," wrote the celebrated artist and educator Elliot Eisner (Eisner, 1996, p. ix), as the configuration of an idea makes possible particular sets of meanings, instructs thought and feeling in particular directions (Eisner, 1972, 1996). In the gestural bridge, we can see how this works. In both situations, it is not hard to see that a sharing of very specific meanings took place which facilitated important personal consequences for the patients.

Interventions of this type call for close observation and for an intimate awareness of the visceral experience of a patient's suffering. This is precisely the kind of contact which is routine in nursing. No one else among the clinical disciplines has our rich access to patients early in the therapeutic process, at a time when the initial clinical goal is, simply, engagement in treatment. Few can achieve our level of intimacy at the earliest stages. Rooted in what nursing theorists have sometimes called an "embodied" or "aesthetic" way of knowing, a general disposition for metaphoric reasoning rather than in scripted technique (Chinn & Kramer, 2014; Chinn & Watson, 1994; Hartrick Doane & Varcoe, 2013; Kagan, Smith, & Chinn, 2014; Stizman & Wright Eichelberger, 2004), gestural bridging enables contact with difficult and isolated patients at a time when other methods of engagement are not available or have not been effective. Metaphoric reasoning is under-reported and under-theorized as a basis for therapeutic communication in nursing. To understand its clinical applications, however, is to expand our understanding of the contents of nursing's therapeutic toolkit. In subsequent chapters, we will examine further examples of this approach and its effects.

References

Akhtar, M. (Ed.). (2011). *Play and playfulness: Developmental, cultural, and clinical aspects.* New York, NY: Jason Aronson.
Ammaniti, M., & Gallese, V. (2014). *The birth of intersubjectivity: Psychodynamics, neurobiology, and the self.* New York, NY: W.W. Norton.
Ammaniti, M., & Stern, D. (1994). *Psychoanalysis and development: Representations and narratives.* New York, NY: New York University Press.
Arieti, S. (1976). *Creativity: The magic synthesis.* New York, NY: Basic Books.
Axline, V. (1969). *Dibs in search of self.* New York, NY: Ballantine Books.

Axline, V. (1974). *Play therapy*. New York, NY: Ballantine Books.

Bollas, C. (2009). *The evocative object world*. New York, NY: Routledge Books.

Bollas, C., & Jemstedt, A. (2011). *The Christopher Bollas reader*. New York, NY: Routledge.

Borbely, A. (2008). Metaphor in psychoanalysis. In R. Gibbs (Ed.), *The Cambridge handbook of metaphor and thought* (pp. 412–424). Cambridge: Cambridge University Press.

Borbely, A. (2013). Metaphor and metonymy as the basis for a new psychoanalytic language. In S. Montana Katz (Ed.), *Metaphor and fields: Common ground, common language, and the future of psychoanalysis* (pp. 79–91). New York, NY: Routledge.

Botella, C., & Botella, S. (2005). *The work of psychic figurability: Mental states without representation*. New York, NY: Routledge.

Botella, C., & Botella, S. (2013). Psychic figurability and unrepresented states. In H. Levine, G. Reed, & D. Scarfone (Eds.), *Unrepresented states and the construction of meaning: Clinical and theoretical contributions* (pp. 95–121). London: Karnac.

Bruner, J., Jolly, A., & Sylva, K. (1976). *Play: Its role in development and evolution*. New York, NY: Basic Books.

Charon, R. (2006). *Narrative medicine: Honoring the stories of illness*. New York, NY: Oxford University Press.

Chinn, P., & Kramer, M. (2014). *Knowledge development in nursing: Theory and process* (9th ed.). New York, NY: Elsevier Mosby.

Chinn, P., & Watson, J. (Eds.). (1994). *Art and aesthetics in nursing*. New York: National League for Nursing Press.

Cienki, A., & Muller, C. (Eds.). (2008). *Metaphor and gesture*. Philadelphia, PA: John Benjamins.

Civitarese, G. (2013). The inaccessible unconscious and reverie as a path to figurability. In H. Levine, G. Reed, & D. Scarfone (Eds.), *Unrepresented states and the construction of meaning: Clinical and theoretical contributions* (pp. 220–239). London: Karnac.

Combs, G., & Freeman, J. (1990). *Symbol, story and ceremony: Using metaphor in individual and family therapy*. New York, NY: W.W. Norton.

Coulson, S. (2008). Metaphor comprehension and the brain. In R. Gibbs (Ed.), *The Cambridge handbook of metaphor and thought* (pp. 177–196). Cambridge: Cambridge University Press.

Donoghue, D. (2014). *Metaphor*. Cambridge, MA: Harvard University Press.

Eckstein, R. (1966). *Children of time and space, of action and impulse*. New York, NY: Meredith Publishing.

Edelman, G., & Tononi, G. (2000). *A universe of consciousness: How matter becomes imagination*. New York, NY: Basic Books.

Eisner, E.W. (1972). *Educating artistic vision*. New York, NY: Macmillan.

Eisner, E.W. (1996). *Cognition and curriculum reconsidered* (2nd ed.). London: Paul Chapman Publishing.

Eliot, T.S. (2001). *The Waste Land*. New York, NY: W.W. Norton.

Erikson, E. (1950). *Childhood and society*. New York, NY: W.W. Norton.

Erikson, E. (1968). *Identity: youth and crisis.* New York, NY: W.W. Norton.

Fauconnier, G., & Turner, M. (2002). *The way we think: Conceptual blending and the mind's hidden complexities.* New York, NY: Basic Books.

Freeman, J., Epston, D., & Lobovits, D. (1997). *Playful approaches to serious problems: narrative therapy with children and their families.* New York, NY: W.W. Norton.

Freud, S. (1953). *On aphasia: A critical study.* New York, NY: International Universities Press.

Freud, S. (1955). *The interpretation of dreams* (J. Strachey, Trans.). New York, NY: Basic Books.

Gerhart, M., & Russell, A. (1984). *Metaphoric process: The creation of scientific and religious understanding.* Fort Worth, TX: Texas Christian University Press.

Gibbs, R.W., Jr. (1994). *The poetics of mind: Figurative thought, language, and understanding.* New York, NY: Cambridge University Press.

Gibbs, R.W., Jr. (Ed.). (2008). *The Cambridge handbook of metaphor and thought.* New York, NY: Cambridge University Press.

Gibbs, R.W., Jr., & Colston, H. (2012). *Interpreting figurative meaning.* New York, NY: Cambridge University Press.

Hartrick Doane, G., & Varcoe, C. (2013). *How to nurse: Relational inquiry with individuals and family in changing health and healthcare contexts.* New York, NY: Wolters Kluwer.

Johnson, M. (1987). *The body in the mind: The bodily basis of reason and imagination.* Chicago, IL: University of Chicago Press.

Johnson, M. (2007). *The meaning of the body: Aesthetics of human understanding.* Chicago, IL: University of Chicago Press.

Kagan, P., Smith, M., & Chinn, P. (2014). *Philosophies and practices of emancipatory nursing: Social justice as praxis.* New York, NY: Routledge.

Katz, S.M. (Ed.) (2013). *Metaphor and fields: Common ground, common language, and the future of psychoanalysis.* New York, NY: Routledge Books.

Keller, H. (2009). *The world I live in and optimism: A collection of essays.* Mineola, NY: Dover Publications.

Koch, S., Fuchs, T., Summa, M., & Muller, C. (Eds.). (2012). *Body memory, metaphor and movement.* Philadelphia, PA: John Benjamins Publishing.

Kopp, R. (1995). *Metaphor therapy: Using client-generated metaphors in psychotherapy.* New York, NY: Brunner-Routledge.

Lakoff, G., & Johnson, M. (1980). *Metaphors we live by.* Chicago, IL: University of Chicago Press.

Lakoff, G., & Nunez, R. (2000). *Where mathematics comes from: How the embodied mind brings mathematics into being.* New York, NY: Basic Books.

Lakoff, G., & Turner, M. (1989). *More than cool reason: A field guide to poetic metaphor.* Chicago, IL: University of Chicago Press.

Landreth, G.L. (2012). *Play therapy: The art of the relationship.* New York, NY: Routledge.

Langer, S. (1953). *Feeling and form: A theory of art.* New York, NY: Charles Scribner's Sons.

Marans, S., Mays, L.C., & Colonna, A.B. (1993). Psychoanalytic views of children's play. In A. Solnit, D. Cohen, & P. Neubauer (Eds.), *The many meanings of play: A psychoanalytic perspective* (pp. 9–28). New Haven, CT: Yale University Press.

Margulis, E.H. (2014). *On repeat: How music plays the mind.* New York, NY: Oxford University Press.

McMullen, L. (2008). Putting in context: Metaphor and psychotherapy. In R. Gibbs (Ed.), *The Cambridge handbook of metaphor and thought* (pp. 397–411). Cambridge: Cambridge University Press.

McNeil, D. (1987). *Psycholinguistics: A new approach.* New York, NY: Harper and Row.

McNeil, D. (1992). *Hand and mind: What gestures reveal about thought.* Chicago, IL: University of Chicago Press.

Modell, A. (2003). *Imagination and the meaningful brain.* Cambridge, MA: MIT Press.

Modell, A. (2013). Metaphor, meaning, and the mind. In S. Montana Katz (Ed.), *Metaphor and fields: Common ground, common language, and the future of psychoanalysis* (pp. 59–66). New York, NY: Routledge Books.

Nattiez, J. (1998). *Music and discourse: Toward a semiology of music.* Princeton, NJ: Princeton University Press.

O'Connor, K., Schaefer, C., & Braverman, L. (2015). *Handbook of play therapy.* New York, NY: Wiley.

Patel, A.D. (2008). *Music, language, and the brain.* New York, NY: Oxford University Press.

Pollio, H., Barlow, E., Fine, M., & Pollio, M. (1977). *Psychology and the poetics of growth.* New York, NY: Lawrence Erlbaum.

Radman, Z. (1997). *Metaphors: figures of the mind.* New York: Kluwer Academic.

Rizzuto, A. (2013). Field theory, the 'talking cure,' and metaphoric processes. In S. Montana Katz (Ed.), *Metaphor and fields: Common ground, common language, and the future of psychoanalysis* (pp. 143–162). New York, NY: Routledge.

Rothenberg, A. (1988). *The creative process of psychotherapy.* New York, NY: W.W. Norton.

Siegelman, E.Y. (1990). *Metaphor and meaning in psychotherapy.* New York, NY: Guilford Press.

Solnit, A., Cohen, D., & Neubauer, P. (1993). *The meaning of play: A psychoanalytic perspective.* New Haven, CT: Yale University Press.

Stern, D. (1985). *The interpersonal worlds of the infant: A view from psychoanalysis and developmental psychology.* New York, NY: Basic Books.

Stizman, K., & Wright Eichelberger, L. (2004). *Understanding the work of nurse theorists: A creative beginning.* New York, NY: Jones and Bartlett.

Thomas, S.P., & Pollio, H.R. (2002). *Listening to patients: A phenomenological approach to nursing research and practice.* New York, NY: Springer Publishing.

Turner, M. (1996). *The literary mind: The origin of thought and language.* New York, NY: Oxford University Press.

Varela, F., Thompson, E., & Rosch, E. (1991). *The embodied mind: Cognitive science and human experience.* Cambridge, MA: MIT Press.

Williams, R.F. (2008). Gesture as a conceptual mapping tool. In A. Cienki & C. Muller (Eds.) *Metaphor and gesture* (pp. 55–92). Philadelphia, PA: John Benjamins Publishing.

Winnicott, D. (2010). *Playing and reality.* New York, NY: Routledge.

Wittgenstein, L. (1980). *Culture and value.* Chicago, IL: University of Chicago Press.

4 Garden-variety analogy

Inpatient psychiatric care facilities often are associated with lovely outdoor spaces. Tree-lined walkways, old oak groves, sprawling grassy lawns, and even working farms are part of the legacy of 19th- and early 20th-century reformers' beliefs about the benefits of fresh air and sunlight and the moral right to haven and asylum. They reflect, as well, the fact that such facilities tended to be built at a remove from bustling commercial urban centers. We nurses don't make the most of this resource, usually because we don't have time, but in part also because we don't think of gardens as part of our own professional toolkit. This is a story that puts a garden at the center of a nurse–patient encounter.

Donald was a strapping young man with a mop of thick black hair and deep brown eyes. Police had brought him to us after he assaulted family members in the apartment they shared and then ransacked a local emergency room, threatening the staff and destroying expensive equipment. He'd been rejected by the multiple care homes to which case managers previously had referred him, the staff there wary of his long-standing record of violence and impulsivity. His chart indicated a lifelong pattern of repeated emergency-room stints, multiple extended hospitalizations, and a diagnostic history almost the size of a reference manual, its length hinting at years of piled-up frustration not only in mental health clinics but also in the offices of school principals and learning specialists.

Within a few days of arrival, Donald had gouged massive crevices in most of the walls, shattered a "break-proof" window panel, and ripped a fire extinguisher box out of its casing. Staff locked him repeatedly in a safety room, separated from other patients, where he deformed door hinges and pulverized walls to chunks in several places. It didn't appear to take much to ignite these rampages, although, as a statistical matter, food figured prominently: one day, another patient intruded in the dinner line; another day, there weren't enough snacks for second helpings;

the kitchen staff ran out of meat loaf; the night-shift staff came in too noisy. "Zero to 100 in five seconds," everybody said, describing the speed of Donald's ascent to fury. From their station in the back, painters and carpenters came to snatch a glance at this young man whose handiwork leaped persistently to the top of every morning's work-order roster.

As medications were started, the nursing staff entered a trial-and-error period of attempting to identify a pattern in Donald's explosions and see what, if anything, we might do to keep our workplace safe. "Show empathy and open-heartedness," they tell you in nursing school. But this wasn't going to come readily, and our first step was decidedly inauspicious: we asked permission to remove Donald's weapons of mass destruction – his heavy shoes – and force him into bare feet.

Unlike many of our more acutely ill patients, Donald had the capacity for apologizing. Within hours of his mayhem, he'd look sad, his head hanging puppy-like. "I'm sorry," he'd say. But even still, he'd remain maddeningly out of contact with himself, unable to articulate a reflective response even to simple questions about his behavior. When we asked him why he'd demolished four nice chairs, for example, or why he'd kicked a bathroom door off its hinges, "I don't know" was all he could muster, in what became an oft-repeated refrain. "I shouldn't have done it. I just want to get out of here."

On the other hand, we could see that Donald cared passionately, in certain perhaps autistic ways, about a wide range of subjects. He not only cared, in fact – he relished. The more we talked to him, the more we learned: he'd read books about astronomy, literature, Greek mythology, the history of world religions. He could recite the Latin names of obscure dinosaurs and describe in detail the principles of air flight, the distances between subway stations, and the workings of the inner ear. Food inspired special passions: he chattered with gusto about grilling, steaming, roasting, and balsamic glaze, about what Turks do with lemons and eggplants and what Italians do with fish. Much of his knowledge came from cookbooks rather than from direct experience. But relating the piney scent of rosemary potatoes and the tangy pop of blueberries on vanilla ice cream, he sparkled. Some of us among the nursing staff were avid home cooks: we delighted in his good moods.

Therapeutic group talk particularly agitated Donald; he wouldn't tolerate any kind of conversation about health, or feelings, or appropriate strategies for behavioral control. He mimicked us with ruthless sarcasm, cursed his physicians and therapists, and stormed out of scheduled programs. "I can't stand this bullshit," he would scream as staff scattered out of spitting distance. "It's the same bullshit every day." So easily triggered, and barred for safety reasons from leaving the locked wing, Donald within a few weeks had managed to trap himself in a familiar cycle of destructiveness, refusal, and the predictable aftermath of penalties and heightened behavioral restrictions. He paced like a caged tiger.

One day, months into his stay and still on strict lock-down, Donald ambled to the nursing station to grab an apple from the counter. "I'm hungry for something to read," he announced, mostly to the air. "And by the way, when's lunch?" The staff at the desk shook their heads and chuckled. "He is such a confused teenager," said an elderly nursing assistant who, in the course of her many decades of work, had raised four children and, now, more than a dozen grandchildren. "He's hungry for everything – books, snacks, knowledge. And then suddenly he remembers he wants to smash us all and break out of here."

For those of us who had raised teenagers, the observation rang instantly true. We glanced around the room, eye contact registering a flash of collective amazement. Donald's erratic behavioral swings indeed seemed to epitomize the characteristic paradox of teenagers: the yearning, on one hand, to take in the wide world, to absorb it and digest it, to make all of it their own – and the craving, on the other hand, to crack everything apart and break free from familiar confines. The furious kicking at walls, the refusal of therapeutic programs, the appetite for food and facts which could be absorbed, digested, and ruminated upon – all these could be "read," in a way, as a gestural communiqué: we had on our hands a pimple-faced teenager in full-throttle contradiction. Most of us have had moments of epiphany at some point in our lives, when some image or idea suddenly emerges to give coherence to what previously had been a jumble. So it was that morning: Donald's pattern of struggle was itself, we decided among ourselves, a clue for some kind of intervention approach. The mothers among us were sure of it.

The benefits of gardens are widely known: the cardiovascular effects of exercise in fresh air, the multisensory pleasures of seeing, smelling, touching, and hearing, the uniquely comforting embrace of sun and soil. There are the emotional and developmental gains to be had from activities combining purposeful aggression with nurturing generosity – that is, digging, chopping, and cutting, alongside watering, fertilizing, and otherwise tending to fragile living things. Trainees in a local horticulturalist program maintained a beautiful garden on grounds adjacent to our building. In luxuriant bloom, it cast through the windows an exuberant mosaic of yellow and pink light. Donald's volatile temper made him ineligible, at this point, to join any group program held in that space. But we nurses speculated that merely getting into the garden, even briefly, might help him express his conflicts more productively.

Taking in the sights and smells, he might engage symbolically – rather than by force – his desire to incorporate the world. Leaving the ward on a regular schedule, in a controlled ritual of exit, might channel his desire to break free from a feeling of confinement. "Similar but safer" was the operating principle with which we took the concept to the clinical leadership. The treating psychiatrist framed the concept as a behavioral intervention: accompanied by a nurse, Donald would be allowed to visit the garden briefly, once a day, staying within the locked gates, following any several-day period that passed without violence.

In the week following this decision, Donald smashed all the ward fire-exit signs and hurled trays across the dining area. But then a few days passed without incident, and despite a prevailing cloud of worry and doubt, I led him out to the garden, watching carefully for pacing, body postures, or facial expressions which might signal impending danger or emotional escalation. Immediately on contact with the breeze and the air, Donald stretched his arms like a lazy cat and stood, blinking and still, in the sunlight.

The first day, we strolled along the walkway and lingered over an area planted with herbs. I plucked a few leaves and offered them. Donald lifted them to his nostrils and inhaled deeply, taking in sage and lavender and lemon-scented geranium. When the horticulturist came out to say hello, Donald cheerfully rattled off the Latin names of at least half a dozen of the ornamentals.

Each of us has a favorite venue for self-expression. Some paint, others play musical instruments. We write, sing, cook, master the basketball court, tinker with small engines. Hobbies such as these give voice to something inside ourselves. So, too, with gardening. Elements of color, texture, fragrance, and composition in gardens evoke memories and ideas much like words in a poem, flavors in a meal, or musical phrases in a symphony. (The green fern in the corner reminds somebody of summer sleep-away camp; the lilac smells vaguely like a grandmother's living room.) The dynamic plot movements of gardens mimic those in theater or literature, as the blooms of late summer, like characters in a novel, retain something of their previous selves when winter arrives, while hinting at what they might, next season, become. Abounding throughout a garden are richness of allegory and allusion and variety in point of view: something shakes like a leaf, irritates like a thorn, withers like violets, or reaches optimistically for the sky, like a sunflower. Shadows are cast; once-new branches finally crumple and curl, losing their vitality. We imagine the sprawling oak embodied in the smallest seedling and find, in spring buds, the promise of impending transfiguration. Who hasn't felt hope for personal renewal in a rosebush on the brink of blooming, or the eerie sense of winter as a reminder that nothing lasts forever? Unencumbered by conventional therapeutic language and released, temporarily, from obligations to relate to others in group settings, Donald, we hoped, might tap this lush narrative resource.

Donald and I strolled in the garden for almost three months, intermittently. We had a pattern: he kicked holes in walls, cracked apart chairs, missed a few days or a week or two of our sessions, depending on the extent of the damage. And then we'd start over, the cycle repeating itself. He listened attentively to the hum of bees and the whistle of breezes; he stroked the soft petals of hibiscus and gingerly traced his fingers along the heart-shaped outlines of *Colocasia* leaves. Parsley and basil and oregano ripened. I snipped fragments for him to taste, triggering lengthy discourses on pasta and soup stock. He identified butterfly species and listed the medicinal uses of *Echinacea*. He sniffed everything with his wide nostrils – the soil, the park bench, a brick wall, his fingernails. Donald did a lot of talking in the garden, and I, mostly, did a lot of standing around. But something began to change.

Occasionally at first, and then more frequently, Donald started pausing. Suspended over a bloom or leaf, turning his ear intently to some object I could not identify, he would stand, almost immobile. Then, after a minute or more, he would launch into a description of someone or something as if it had been called up, that moment, to memory. Increasingly, over time, these were personal stories rather than recitations of fact. He told me about a grandmother born in the Greek Isles, a social worker he once knew, a book his mother used to read to him, a fairy tale he remembered. Without probing for information about context or implications, I could not identify the meanings of the associations the garden was conjuring, the thoughts which might be linked to whatever stream of images it had released. But I could see that Donald was beginning to make contact with a narrator inside himself.

Gradually, with setbacks which became less frequent as the weeks passed, Donald's violent outbursts tapered. Then one day, a fight broke out among some other patients. Instead of entering the fray, as he might have done earlier, Donald stepped back and removed himself, reminding himself out loud, "I should stay out of this." It was a benchmark moment – our first explicit signal that he had begun to show a capacity for regulatory self-talk.

Everyone working with Donald agreed, in the days following this episode, that Donald had responded well to medication and was growing more comfortable, and, moreover, that the garden routine had played a role in his progress. He was soon released from the most onerous behavioral restrictions and enabled to move around more freely in the building and on the grounds. He began joining scheduled programs and was signed on to one-on-one counseling sessions, a change he now welcomed. He attached himself to a social group of similar-aged peers. His schedule filled. We scaled back our walks as other activities and relationships took precedence and seemed, by that point, far more valuable and important to him.

It was a long time before anyone felt Donald was safe enough even to be considered for transfer to a less restrictive setting. There was no magic in his progress. But a year of intensive interdisciplinary work passed, during which a charming, vibrant, and often funny young man emerged, a young man who had allowed many new people into his circle. And finally the day came when he waved at the door, dragging a rather hilariously heavy bag of books and clothing to the next, hopefully better, chapter of his life.

The garden as a bridge

What might be said, looking back, about the nursing intervention described here? As with the activities described in previous chapters, it embodied many of the traditional nursing values and competencies – patience, perseverance, caring, consistency, reliability, confidence, generosity, optimism. We gave these in abundance – and over a great span of time. Equally importantly, however, is that the nursing team took seriously, particularly in the beginning, the communicative content of Donald's violent gestures; we looked and listened before dismissing his bizarre, frightening behaviors merely as symptoms needing to be contained or managed. We engaged the details of Donald presentations as ideas which might be thought about and transformed to productive use.

It is worth noting that we made no particularly dramatic show of attentiveness and compassionate care. Nobody talked to Donald about his feelings. Nobody tried to support him to achieve formal or conventional conscious insight. Nobody praised him for participating in a therapeutic activity or offered words of comfort or support for his obvious suffering. The opposite, in fact, was true, since Donald had come to us uniquely unable to tolerate traditional therapeutic "talk" and was intensely hostile to any interactional format which triggered even slight feelings of being boxed in.

Rather, a playful ritual itself did the therapeutic work. The game of going outdoors, of exit and return, was our way of "speaking" to Donald, without words, about the feeling of yearning for release and being free from a plaguing confinement. The sensory stimulations of the garden, meanwhile, offered an indirect vocabulary of plenty – a richness of scents and sights – that suggested, analogically, the wide world Donald seemed so eager to master and absorb. The activity allowed us to cast representational structure around themes for which Donald had no language, inviting him to experience these in a simple, bodily way, before he had mastered any capacity for explicit self-reflection and spoken vocabulary that might more conventionally express them. This was the conceptual "mapping" which facilitated his transition toward an ultimately successful engagement in more formal therapeutic modalities.

5 The house as a grammatical form

Valerie was a middle-aged woman with a lifelong history of alcohol and drug abuse. Her adult years had been marked by multiple acute and long-term hospitalizations, repeated episodes of extreme violence, and removal from supervised residential homes in several different cities. She had been diagnosed with schizoaffective disorder. After running away from a group care home and assaulting customers at a gas station, she was committed again to a locked facility for evaluation and treatment.

For eight months, Valerie screamed through the night. She kicked staff members and patients who approached her and scratched the aides who attempted bathing and hygiene assistance. She stripped off clothing, knocked over furniture, "painted" windows with feces and soap, and spent many nights in a special safety room separated from the general patient sleeping area. Placed on close monitoring for her own protection as well as that of others, she grew increasingly socially isolated as a discouraged staff began avoiding serious engagement with her. She was transferred to a unit specializing in neurodegenerative disorders, where programming and milieu structure centered on sensory support. But even in the new setting, Valerie made no progress. Episodically, she refrained from screaming while allowing one or two staff to shower her, wash her hair, or help her put on her clothes. Outside these brief interactions, she remained hostile and regressed; attempts to initiate conversation were met with aggression or silence.

At one point, Valerie was transferred to a general medical hospital following an infection and an acute medication reaction. Ripping out intravenous lines and breaking a staff member's fingers, she was deemed to be unmanageable and soon returned for psychiatric care. Our clinical team brainstormed what might be done while her medical and lab status stabilized. Other than the violence reported in her medical chart, we knew little about her life, and since she didn't speak in whole sentences, she remained, for a long time, a mystery. One evening, however, she forced her way out of the supervision of a nursing assistant, ran down a hallway, and grabbed a small doll belonging to another patient.

This was the first time we'd seen Valerie show interest in any specific object external to herself. Doll play, as is widely known, has a long history in child psychotherapy, where it enables children to project thoughts and feelings too complex for their limited vocabularies. Observers have noted that doll play can provide sensory stimulation and comfort for older adults in dementia-care settings. We found no reports about the use of doll play with adult psychiatric inpatients. But we embraced the possibility that Valerie's behavior might be key to some kind of activity which finally could engage her. After much deliberation, the team came to an agreement, and nurses mobilized. One of us bought in one of our children's old dollhouses and a set of wooden furniture pieces. Another donated a miniature plastic "family" and an assortment of tiny household objects such as lamps, pillows, and blankets. We added a few small plush puppies and kittens and set up a table in an activity room.

In light of Valerie's history of anxiety related to staff-initiated verbal communications, we opted for a non-directive approach – bringing her to the activity room a few times a week, presenting the materials one by one, silently, with no direction or guidance, and seeing what might happen. We wanted to give Valerie maximal freedom to create her own themes and modulate in her own way the relational experience with supervising staff. Working closely with us to develop a monitoring protocol for tracking Valerie's progress, the unit psychiatrist initiated new medication trials as the nursing team launched yet another attempt to make contact.[1]

Two staff members flanked Valerie on the first day – ready to respond if she bolted. But it turned out that we didn't need to worry. From the moment she entered the activity room and noticed the play materials on the table, Valerie was hooked. Her interest was intense. In the first play sessions, she accepted only the plush animals and a few pieces of the furniture, pushing away any offers of the human figurines. She took chairs, tables, sinks, and stoves and piled them, one after the other, in bizarre, chaotic mounds in the corners of several rooms. But her grasp on the plush animals was tender and deliberate – with the tips of her fingers – as she placed each one on the shelves. In stunningly clearly articulated sentences, she assigned each one a name. "This is Anthony's dog," she said. "This is Raymond's brown puppy." We were shocked.

Few staff on the unit had previously heard Valerie speak in whole sentences, and none of us knew who Anthony and Raymond were, as their names appeared nowhere in her chart history. Nonetheless, the names and identities which Valerie assigned in these early sessions remained intact throughout the subsequent months, and Valerie referenced them repeatedly in the story lines which unfolded as the intervention progressed.

The second week, rather than merely naming and identifying characters, Valerie started arranging plausible activity scenes in which characters were depicted as active agents. She organized the animals in a circle around a table, for example, and said "this is my birthday party." She began accepting the human figurines and adding them to the arrangements. In the third and fourth weeks, her originally bizarre, seemingly haphazard piles of furniture gave way to increasingly visually orderly and logically coherent compositions. She aligned all the chairs in neat rows along the wall edges, for example, and separated out functionally plausible two- and three-item settings of tables with objects such as flowerpots, food bowls, and lamps. Her story lines expanded to include more than one sentence and more complex narrative structures. She saw a box of yellow plastic blocks in a corner of the activity room, for example, and stood up to fetch it. Arranging the blocks delicately in a yellow pile on one of the shelves, she described an ambulance rescue in which a puppy disappeared while she and her mother were saved from a house fire. ("The puppy dog sleeps when Anthony sleeps...The doggy got lost in a fire. I don't know what happened to him"). She also identified a purported future husband ("This is Rocky. I am going to marry him") and referenced a character, Susan, not represented by any object, who "drives the ambulance that saves mommy's life and my life." One day, after painstakingly sorting the furniture collection by size – large objects in one pile and small ones in another – she neatly balanced all the smaller pieces on top of the larger ones, forming a double-decker row. "I am old enough to take care of my own kids," she said.

In the fourth week, Valerie had an aggressive outburst. After all the furniture was arranged, she took in her hand a small bookcase and began slamming it, first on one shelf and then on the next, screaming repeatedly, "I do not want Daddy here!" She then grabbed other furniture pieces off the shelves and threw them across the room. Following this, in the fifth week, she began, for the first time, organizing multiple simultaneous narrative scenes in different parts of the house. One play session, she arranged all the "children" and "infants" together in one room with the bed and the armchairs (a scene she called "babysitting") while, in the adjacent space, she seated all the "adults" in chairs lining the back wall, explaining "this is me in group." Just before the two-month mark, Valerie arranged what she called "group home" scenes and scenes of mothers and children. In one session, she spent many minutes tenderly arranging a plush bear's clothing as she tucked the bear into "bed" and adjusted its blanket. She talked about her mother and some shopping trips they had taken together.

As the visual coherence and narrative complexity of her doll play increased over time, Valerie's behavior on the unit also evolved. She no longer needed sedating medication or close staff monitoring; her physical and verbal aggression slowed and then stopped. Staff reported Valerie was attending most unit programming, sleeping in her regular bedroom, and joining other patients at mealtimes. She had begun initiating conversations, asking comprehensible questions about scheduling and snacks. She agreed to showers and began cooperating with phlebotomy and clinic appointments such as podiatry. She even gave one of us a "gift" of a small stuffed animal she had stored in her bedroom. "I want you to have this," she said, revealing what seemed to us to be a new awareness of the feelings of others. "I think you might like it." Valerie was stabilized on a new medication regimen at this time as well, and we marveled, as an interdisciplinary team, at the transformations which accompanied this convergence of pharmacological and non-medication-based therapeutic interventions. There was a brightness, an optimism, about the Valerie who had awakened before our eyes, and all of us were enjoying it, and enjoying her.

Around the eighth week, something changed abruptly. Valerie came to the activity room eagerly, as before. But one morning, she didn't talk about the figurine arrangements or tell any of their stories. Rather, her configurations were purely decorative – ornamental rather than narrative: "That looks pretty," she said, placing teddy bears in each corner of the dollhouse. "Nice." Valerie had not described anything previously in this way, and we took it as a signal: I told Valerie I was going to put the dollhouse away for a while, and she agreed. Her schedule was full by then of other, more conventional group programs and therapies. For the first time since her admission, Valerie was permitted to leave the locked unit independently to visit the snack shop and go to the gym without staff supervision. It was not long afterward that she was finally able to leave the locked facility with confidence, dignity, and some measure of restored capacity for self-determination and self-care.

Structure as a bridge toward grammar

On the surface, our dollhouse game was ordinary play – something fun for the patient to do, something that might keep her busy. Like most good nursing interventions, it involved creating a safe and empathic interactional milieu, a relational environment characterized by consistency, reliability, predictability, and structured routine. It called for sensitivity and patience, and so on, on the part of the nurse. It had, in other words, many of the typical characteristics of good nursing communication. But in its deeper logical structure, the game contained something else which was equally important. Embedded inside it was a metaphorical reference to the congruence between inside space and outside space – a suggestion about ideas held inside receiving form and expressive structure from an external physical source. Taking up the analogy, enacting it through play, Valerie moved a step toward rediscovering her own capacity for narrativity.

A century ago, the linguist Roman Jakobson noted links between geometry and grammar – between external shape structures and visual compositional forms, on one hand, and, on the other hand, the internal structures of speech and thought (Jakobson, 1987). It can be said that our nursing intervention exemplified this principle. Establishing a venue in which Valerie could assert control and decision-making, but with materials of interest to her, doll play provided an open-ended "dialect" by which she could disentangle, quite literally, some of the story elements of her life – assemble and arrange them, stand apart, observe, and consider them. The dollhouse, we might say, became an external grammar as its concrete shape offered an ad hoc structure for calling up and organizing meanings from the background noise of experience.

Our doll activity did not emerge from a manual of nursing interventions or list of formal objectives read off from a diagnostic chart. But it activated the patient's capacity for observational and narrative agency during a period when conventional words were not available to her, even though, quite clearly, she had something significant to say. Doll play offered a transitional configuration which linked a complex internal mental experience to a simpler, more externally share-able structure for representing and exchanging meaning. Moreover, it illustrated the success which can result from intensive interdisciplinary collaboration. We hoped, as Valerie left, that she would be able to access consistent and reliable community supports and sustain a life for herself free from confinement and institutionalization, and that she would continue, when the feeling moved her, to play.

Note

1 Some of the material in this section has appeared previously, in different form, in Birnbaum, S., Hanchuk, H., & Nelson, M. (2015). Therapeutic doll play in the treatment of a severely impaired psychiatric inpatient: dramatic

clinical improvement with a non-traditional nursing intervention. *Journal of Psychosocial Nursing and Mental Health Services* 53 (5), 22–27. Reprinted with permission from SLACK Inc.

References

Fauconnier, G. & Turner, M. (2002). *The way we think: Conceptual blending and mind's hidden complexities.* New York, NY: Basic Books.

Jakobson, R. (1987). *Language in literature.* Cambridge, MA: Harvard University Press.

Lakoff, G. & Johnson, M. (1999). *Philosophy in the flesh: The embodied mind and its challenge to Western thought.* New York, NY: Basic Books.

6   Rhythms and regularities in a musical bridge

Medics wheeled the ambulance gurney through the admissions gate and locked it into position, releasing Aaron's wrists from the restraint straps. Aaron hoisted his body to standing, blinked under the hall lamp, and lunged for the doctor's throat, clenching tightly. Staff shouted for help. Aaron had to be tied to the restraint chair twice that first afternoon and then again the following day. Word got around: the new patient is big and out of control. The unit's clinical and administrative leaders announced an emergency meeting as the nurses closed off doors in an office-wing hallway, creating, in effect, a cocoon of locked space where Aaron could pace back and forth without hurting any of the more fragile patients.

This was the epitome, to our minds, of an interagency disconnect. More than six feet tall, weighing nearly 300 pounds, possessing, evidently, only a smattering of words, Aaron presented with a dual diagnosis – psychiatric conditions co-occurring with intellectual and developmental disabilities. He lived all his life previously in the care of his mother and father, who'd supported dressing, bathing, eating, toileting, and so on – the multitude of daily tasks Aaron couldn't perform alone. But Aaron's aging and increasingly infirm and frail parents could no longer find the strength to care for this complicated, physically demanding and now 30-something year-old son. It was a story achingly familiar in the human-services business: transitions taken the hard way.

Prior to his admission, Aaron had been placed on a regional "priority" list awaiting assignment to residential housing, as case workers scrambled to identify open bed space among the limited group which specialized in care for severely developmentally disabled adults. The first referral rejected Aaron, as did the second, staff noting that psychiatric comorbidities and a history of aggression rendered him a risk to their other residents. A facility finally was found which would accept him, but in the unfamiliar setting, Aaron fared poorly. He stopped eating, refused bathing or changes of clothing, smashed down a door, urinated on the floor, shattered glass windows, and yanked a staff member to the ground, ripping out clumps of her hair. Staff noted a tendency to pace irritably and hold his left hand to his ear, as if soothing an earache or listening to a voice. There were multiple back-and-forth transfers over subsequent weeks to a local emergency room. Clinicians agreed: Aaron was not tolerating medications normally prescribed to manage aggression or psychotic symptoms. He needed, for the time being, a more intensive level of care.

And so it came to pass that a lumbering, wordless young man, gripped by terror and drenched in urine and feces, without his parents and torn from the comforts of a home he'd known all his life, was strapped by the wrists and ankles to an ambulance gurney and delivered to the front door.

Estimates vary on the proportion of people with intellectual and developmental disabilities who experience co-occurring psychiatric disorders, but studies suggest it might be as many as a third (Quintero & Flick, 2010). In administration and funding, the mental health system has operated separately, historically, from the system of services for intellectual and developmental disabilities. On both sides of the institutional gap, agency staff feel ill equipped to provide adequate services for clients with multiple complex needs, as care protocols and treatment providers specialize, for the most part, in one set of issues or the other. Within each system of care, personnel tend to expect the other to provide services. Aaron exemplified, it seemed, the dually diagnosed patient who "falls between the cracks" – whose multifaceted needs seem to surpass the capacity of any single institution or agency to address them.

The records accompanying Aaron were sparse at first, further complicating our initial efforts to determine what, exactly, had been "done" in the past which was helpful to him and what, based on experience, we might avoid repeating. To what programs or treatment protocols, now, might we safely assign him? The chart history indicated a hodge-podge of diagnoses: a mood disorder, an anxiety disorder, autism, among others. Other than these, we knew little. Watching Aaron's anxious pacing, his compulsive restlessness, his obvious suffering, we struggled to define clear clinical treatment goals – the formal objectives which serve as a starting point for intervention decisions. Regarding his baseline pattern of functioning and personal strengths, we knew essentially nothing. What, in such a case, could be the clinical target for our work? The nurses wrote a traditional care plan: hygiene, nutrition, safety, routine assessment, medication compliance, and so on. But how could such a plan get started? Nobody could get near this man without a significant struggle.

Records trickled in. A social worker invested overtime in myriad interagency emails and managed eventually to engage Aaron's parents by phone. Years previously, we learned, he had graduated from a special school. He'd shown interest in puzzles and building blocks and was well liked by teachers and peers, though his spoken vocabulary, at its peak, had never included more than a few words. Later, as a young adult, he had attended a well-regarded day program, exercised in a gym, and even, for a time, held a paid job sorting containers in a training center. His condition had declined as his parents' advancing debility turned into a cascade of personal disruptions, derailing long-standing life routines. We saw little evidence now of Aaron's previous level of functioning. So we reached, at first, for familiar and available tools.

Aaron shoved aside the picture board which language-limited patients sometimes use as a communication aid to point to what they need (the picture of a bathroom, for example, or a bed, or a plate of food). He snubbed ball play, ring toss, and even simple puzzles arranged on a table, angrily scattering pieces to the floor. Pop music, a perennial favorite for most patients, sent him storming truculently down the hall, swiping at his ears as if waving away flies. He made no eye contact, acknowledged no greeting, said nothing, and he responded to no toileting or hygiene prompts. Several of the mental health techs sustained bruises within the first few days trying to change Aaron's filthy clothing and wash him. His monitoring status was upgraded to the highest level so that he could be observed by multiple staff at the same time, as one of the psychologists initiated a strict behavioral regimen – praise and snacks for any move toward cooperation with basic care. Between the locked office doors, the hallway reeked. It was not hard to miss Aaron's almost unfathomable isolation – an exile from fundamental structures of self-care and social exchange. By trial and error, however, some intrepid evening-shift staff found that if they occupied both his hands simultaneously with juice and cookies, Aaron could hold still for just long enough to accept oral medications and allow for his brow and cheeks to be wiped briefly with a washcloth. So began, inauspiciously, Aaron's physical care. We tiptoed around him, guarded and vigilant.

From the shift hand-off, we knew that Aaron paced the hallway nearly continuously, from early morning until late at night. From one edge of the closed-off wing to the other, he treaded along the wall edges with an almost metronomic relentlessness, single-mindedly, aggressively pushing away anyone who stood in the path of this compulsive motion. The clinical team reviewed the nursing reports with desperation every shift, searching for signs of a landing point on the lunar surface of this implacable restlessness.

Rhythm saturates social life, Henri Lefebvre, the French philosopher, has written (Lefebvre, 2004). It infuses our work and our play, our encounters with traffic and taxes and school calendars, our sleep cycles and eating schedules, our contact with nature and our contact with people. Rhythmic patterns are inscribed as a fundamental constituent of identity, reverberating in our oldest memories and fundamental sense of self. So when a rhythmic order is taken away, our bodies continue, distantly, to hear it, and we attempt, perhaps unwittingly, to reconstitute it.

The English romantic poet William Wordworth is considered the master of poetic rhythm, his huge body of work dense with a spare oscillating murmur, a determinacy that replicates, in sound, the rhythmicity of a walk in the countryside. It is said of Wordsworth that he wandered perhaps 180,000 miles in the course of his long life. His sister wrote in her diaries of the compulsiveness and single-mindedness with which he traversed, in thundering rain or in blistering heat, the small yard outside the cottage they shared (Gros, 2011).

Walking has long been associated with talking – the rhythms of steady step-wise motion bonded with the dance of voices summoning meaning in turns. Two and a half millennia ago, Aristotle founded a school of philosophy known to us as "the peripatetic" – named after the ancient Greek word *peripatein*, which means to walk and to converse, to engage in a dialogue while walking. We marveled, now, at Aaron's ravenous, unending conversation of one foot in front of the other. Nightly, wobbling from exhaustion and heavily sedating medications, he collapsed into a mattress we'd placed on the floor for him. The staff covered him with blankets as he slept, tucking around the edges tenderly, pushing sweaty hair off his forehead and gazing in fearful wonder.

Psychotherapy's aim, in general, is to teach self-talk – to help people grow a capacity for thoughtful internal dialogue. Words are chosen, ideas shared. Over time, the practice lessons between therapist and patient are internalized. And if all goes well, what was outside grows inside: the patient learns to initiate a dialogue with his own mind, to think things through. Nurses feel this keenly in our own professional version of it: we have all, at one time or another, felt the way our resolute and generous presence grows in our patients enduring feelings of solidity and security – feelings of maternal care which they absorb and learn to summon up themselves if our interventions are successful. But Aaron presented what seemed like the converse: here was a young man locked already in a rigid back and forth – a compulsive conversational motion so savagely rigorous as to be almost impenetrable. To reinsert into this lockstep oscillation the softening cadence of an external human voice – this felt to all of us to be the task at hand. But how does one enter a conversation with someone who is closed off to words? We didn't know. So we monitored carefully for response to medications, supported hygiene and nutrition to whatever extent we could, and waited for an idea to make itself known.

Pablo Casals, the Spanish cellist, was only 13 years old when he stumbled on a yellowed package of old sheet music in a tiny thrift shop in Barcelona. It turned out to be Johann Sebastian Bach's cello suites, six short works originally written around 1720 but subsequently mostly neglected, as musicians of the 18th and early 19th centuries considered them dry and overly mathematical, something like practice exercises. Casals fell in love with them, and, in 1936, when he was 60 years old and already world-renowned, finally recorded them. Their popularity soared, and today they are considered among the most profoundly elegant and poignant works in the classical repertoire. (One of them was played at the opening of New York City's World Trade Center memorial.) There are six of these suites, each organized symmetrically, with the harmonic precision and rigor for which Bach is famous, and each divided into six symmetrical smaller sections. Like other music of their time, they are polyphonic, which means a multiplicity of voice lines calls out in twining layers as the work progresses, evoking a sound image of depth and dialogic exchange.

Musically, the cello suites convey the idea of a voice in plaintive conversation with itself. Composer Tod Machover (2007) tells us that the cello, among all orchestral instruments, is the one which comes the closest in range to the human voice – its lowest notes at the bottom of the basso profundo, its top ranges capable of something like the trilling of the highest soprano. I had been listening in my car on the way to work. My mind called up suddenly a comment by one of the nursing aides: "Maybe he likes classical?" Aaron's psychiatrist embraced the idea. What did we have to lose, after all, from introducing our patient to Bach?

A few of us assembled in an office cubicle to load the material, huddled like co-conspirators around the unit MP3 player. Briefly in the morning, then at mid-day, and then again in the late afternoon, for short bouts, Bach's elegant cello suites called down the hallway, odd notes trickling every so often through the narrow slits in the doorway out to the general patient area. Aaron did not swat them away, as he had done with other music. On the contrary: we saw from the beginning that he paused, turning his head, at first quizzically, to listen. After a few sessions of this, we gave him a chair and noted a brief serenity with which he sat himself down quietly, listening for some minutes before resuming his anxious pacing. It was, unmistakably, contact.

Over the next few weeks, an interdisciplinary team played the cello suites intermittently, at least once but usually several times a day, each time introducing new activities or milieu elements to the backdrop of their musical accompaniment. Aaron allowed himself to stand at a table as the cello spoke around him. He permitted one staff member to escort him to the bathroom, another to wash him. His restless pacing began to diminish, as he paused more frequently, and, over a period of days, he began responding to simple directions ("go wash your hands," "sit here for lunch") which previously had greatly irritated him. Hoping to activate whatever reserve of words might resurface from Aaron's mysterious silence, the floor-duty staff began narrating each increment of advance: "You changed your pants!" "You used the toilet!" "You are sitting in the chair!" Aaron began pointing – to a blanket, to the toilet, to the bed, to a paper towel – initiating goal-directed communications. He agreed to play a ball game. He worked a puzzle. Slowly, with the music shepherding his emergence from isolation, he accepted many of the activities which initially had been angrily refused. Three weeks in, we re-opened the hall doors so Aaron could enter the general patient area for brief forays around the nursing station. The cello suites attracted converts: more than a handful of staff members downloaded them for personal use.

As Aaron grew more comfortable, happier and more relaxed, engaging more readily in conventional therapeutic activities with the psychology and rehab departments, and so on, and allowing more of the clinical staff into his circle of contact, we turned off the music. A warm, good-natured, and likeable personality emerged over the course of the ensuing month, and Aaron was able, finally, to transition to a richer and far less restrictive community setting.

Rhythm metaphors

What can be said about this strange episode? First, that it exemplified interdisciplinary collaboration and mutual respect on the part of diverse members of a clinical team. This is rarer than we like to admit in healthcare, and its importance cannot be overstated. Nurses:

cherish those moments of genuine collaboration whenever they make an appearance. Second, that nurses played a crucial role, particularly in the beginning, as care was being initiated. Our close-range observations and round-the-clock monitoring created a picture of the patient as a person, with a style and disposition and preferences of his own, rather than a chart entry. Third, that it involved optimism, perseverance, compassion, a capacity for sensitivity and forgiveness, and a willingness to try something new – core nursing values. But in addition to these, the intervention contained, as well, the analogical structure described elsewhere in this book. Trapped at first in a communicative idiom which took the form of compulsive walking, Aaron was able to encounter in the cello's textured counterpoint an oscillating rhythmicity, highly personal and familiar perhaps in a certain uncanny respect, but which allowed him to enter into communication with something outside his own suffering. Tender in its tones and firm in its structures – evocative or reminiscent, possibly, of something in Aaron's previous family life – the vocal dialect of the cello enabled us to elaborate viscerally with him the ideas of regularity, communicative reciprocity, and orderly human exchange. We had found Bach almost by accident, by the luck of my having had a CD collection in the glove box of my car. But in this music of a particular texture and rhythm and color, we had identified a means for connecting to this otherwise almost impossibly distant young man.

"Little as we know about the way in which we are affected by form, by colour, and light," wrote Florence Nightingale in 1859, "we do know this, that they have an actual physical effect" (Nightingale, 1859). The gestural bridge here – in music form – speaks to this long-standing but underutilized nursing concept. We hoped that Aaron would find friends, safety, pleasure, and purpose in his new place of residence, and that music would continue to inspire and comfort him.

References

Gros, F. (2011). *A philosophy of walking*. New York, NY: Verso.

Lefebvre, H. (2004). *Rhythmanalysis: Space, time and everyday life*. London: Continuum.

Machover, T. (2007). My cello. In S. Turkle (Ed.), *Evocative objects: Things we think with* (pp. 14–21). Cambridge, MA: MIT Press.

Nightingale, F. (1859). *Notes on nursing: What it is, what it is not*. New York, NY: D. Appleton. Retrieved from www.digital.library.upenn.edu/women/nightingale/nursing.html

Quintero, M., & Flick, S. (2010). Co-occurring mental illness and developmental disabilities. *Social Work Today* 10(5), 6.

7   Nursing knowledge and nursing art: implications for learning and professional development[1]

Years after my patient Donald was discharged from inpatient care (see Chapter 4), a young girl attempted to hang herself with a hair band on an adolescent unit where I was working. An aide found her and cut the string, and we were able, thankfully, to revive her. Administrative and clinical leadership responded quickly to the episode, with sensitivity and compassion, offering counseling and paid days off to anyone who had participated in the rescue. I appreciated the exemplary "trauma-informed" response. But I found it, at the same time, strangely diminishing.

Rather than being engaged as an object of compassion, I would have preferred in that moment to explore some more complicated and challenging subjects than my personal feelings – recent staffing reductions, for instance, the condition of the emergency equipment, gaps in the clinical team's prior communications about the patient, and the perennial tensions, in any mental health setting, between the risks inherent in hair bands and earrings and the rights of patients to keep personal possessions. All these are familiar to the seasoned nurse. So the "care" talk felt to me, at that time, like a kind of taming – a caging of my own subjective reaction. I found myself thinking back to Donald, and I noted, in retrospect, how our initial insistence on displays of nursing care and "compassion" – the standard, well-honed tools of our trade – might have felt to him like an engulfing kind of confinement. So it was that my own experience, linked in my thoughts to Donald's, led me to rethink the nature of nursing interventions.

If your only tool is a hammer, the saying goes, everything looks like a nail. So, too, with nursing's conception of what it means to communicate therapeutically. Nurses are trained in verbal techniques of therapeutic communication – repeating, summarizing, paraphrasing, validating, and so on. We are trained, as well, in compassionate body language – in showing openness and attentiveness though position, posture, tone, facial expression, and the like. But *being attentive* is not the same as *paying attention*. Displays of compassion and attentive care are an important and valuable part of our work, but they are not the same, logically and conceptually, as the more intellectually rigorous task of attuning to what might be specific, distinctive, and unique in a patient's subjective categories of thought and experience.

Gestural bridge activities – the metaphoric representations which I have described in this book – are a form of communication which begins not with prior assumptions about the care or compassion our patients might need, or with ready-made manuals about "correct" methods for displaying them. Rather, the activities described here emerge from a far more complex source – a unity of reason and imagination, feeling and thought – which philosopher Mark Johnson has called "imaginative rationality" (Johnson, 1987) and which many writers in the psychoanalytic tradition have long identified as a core of creative therapeutic work (Arieti, 1976; Borbely, 2008; Modell, 2003; Rothenberg, 1988). Elliot Eisner, a painter who became one of the leading educational theorists of the last century, noted that literacy comes in many shapes and sizes; to support someone to become literate means to grow the capacity to encode and decode meanings constructed across the great variety of forms which humans use to represent the contents of our consciousness (Eisner, 1996). A related claim might be made for nursing: it involves a multiplicity of literacies, some of them having to do with cultivating imagination and metaphorical reasoning as a means for exploring and evaluating new possibilities for patients.

What lessons might be harbored in the stories here regarding the ways we are educated to be professional nurses, the ways we sensitize our ears to patients' voices and learn to reach inside ourselves for connections and associations not previously articulated? How might nurses promote this more "poetic" mode of understanding (Gibbs, 1994) so that it can be brought more consistently to bedside practice? I suggest, in this chapter, a few general principles. These are not so much about skills or specific knowledge content as about overall orientation and disposition. They are a way of looking at things.

The centrality of the body

The first and most important principle relates to the centrality of the body in nursing consciousness, a lesson which was driven home to me by my patient Wendy. Wendy had been homeless, intermittently, for much of her adult life. Sleeping on the street appealed to her because of the relative independence it afforded compared with institutionalization or supervised group residency. But every so often, during periods of increased personal stress the origins of which were unknown to us, she'd be found wandering in dark alleys or cowering in corners, mumbling, under-dressed for cold weather, her hair and clothing caked with feces and reeking of urine, her fingernails long as eagle talons. Patients like Wendy are known in the business, pejoratively, as "frequent flyers" – they enter and exit through a revolving door of repeating discharges and readmissions.

At the point of Wendy's re-hospitalizations, nurses would get saddled with the order to wash her – by force if necessary. Anyone who has bathed a homeless, incontinent, and grossly psychotic patient knows well the hazards. Combative resistance in a slippery, wet room can be frightening and dangerous both for the patient and for the nurse. But to get into a shower room with Wendy was to realize the principle which Florence Nightingale, in her 1859 classic *Notes on Nursing* (Nightingale, 1859), placed at the core of our profession: that the body itself is the source of understanding and communication, the ultimate repository for every way we know and tell. Wendy wailed like a banshee about Nazi gas chambers, rendering achingly clear, as I restrained her, the degree to which she was living the suffering of her concentration-camp-survivor parents. Her rage at my offers of fresh clothing and a diaper ("Don't waste a new one, you stupid cunt!") cast into high relief her punishing self-explorations about the nature of entitlement and waste in a world of suffering and deprivation – the question of how much might be too much for one person to ask. Wendy raised her fists to punch me when I offered to clean and trim her fingernails, as she swore she had been using them as can openers. An obviously delusional statement on its surface, it gave poignant reflection to the quandary she had posited between her own body and the rest of the world: what does it mean to survive and "make do" in a place where resources are scarce, where there is cruelty and absence and want?

At the advanced level, psychiatric nursing increasingly consists of practices divorced from body experience: we dispense prescriptions for psychotropic medications to be administered by others, we take seminars in leadership and management and pile certifications alongside our titles. At the level of the floor-duty nurse, meanwhile, staffing shortages and burgeoning documentation and paperwork demands mean that physical care tasks – once the nurse's domain – fall, increasingly, to nursing assistants and support technicians. This is moving our profession in the wrong direction – away from the direct relational work at the core of good nursing.

Patients such as Wendy, Joe, Valerie, and Aaron remind us that the body remains the mediator of mental experience – the source of its uniquely terrifying and remarkable metaphoric language. To communicate with persistently mentally ill patients such as these requires a willingness, first and foremost, to return to the original and foundational source of nursing understanding. It requires caring for patients in personal, somatic ways. Nursing understanding begins, we see in all the encounters described here, with palpable physicality. It is knowledge of the body, of a specific body, and intimacy with that specific body's unique voices.

Embracing the many forms of language

Which brings us to the second principle – about taking seriously the potential meaning-content of patients' bodily gestures and behaviors, encountering respectfully and not dismissively the great diversity of narrative forms in which people might be telling stories.

Norton, my patient, rolled on the ground in a bizarre, grotesquely disturbing manner – a perverse choreography of slow-motion contortions. He crawled, coiled, twisted. His taut, trim body had the persistence of a wind-up toy: finding himself in a corner, he'd switch direction. This behavior made him an easy target for other patients' frustrations and anger – a temptation made all the worse by his mumbling in a gibberish nobody understood. We nurses did our best to keep him clean and fed. We monitored for bruises and exhausted all means to engage him to sit still, especially when visitors or inspectors came, as his ridiculous prone displays made it seem we were neglectful. There had been months of medication trials and evaluations by neurologists and specialists in catatonia and other extreme schizophrenia manifestations. Still, he crawled like a snake on the floor.

Kevin was about the same age as Norton; they'd known each other for years. This is an interesting fact about psychiatric care: inpatient and outpatient programs and facilities, short-term and long-term, voluntary and forced, public and private, are organized geographically into a regional system of care, so cohorts of chronically and persistently ill patients often run into one another repeatedly across multiple settings over periods of time. A social history evolves between them which transcends any specific episode of treatment or institutionalization. Kevin approached me angrily one evening as I struggled to coax Norton out of a puddle of chicken in which he was twisting on the dining-area floor.

"I myself had once been afflicted," Kevin began. Kevin had been a "subway prophet" – the kind of aggressively religiously preoccupied

patient, well known in urban psychiatric nursing, who frightens commuters with intrusive preaching on the train platform and makes mothers grasp their children closer.

"I myself had felt the darkness of the soul. I myself was drowned in
the depths of the sea. I myself was like the worm and the snake, without
the strength to walk and the breath to speak."

"Okay," I said. "What's up?"

"Don't you know what he's saying to you?" Kevin hissed, pointing to
his old acquaintance in the puddle. "Just look at his shoulders! Look at
how they squeeze together! Can't you see he's squeezing his heart? Can't
you see he's showing you how much it hurts?"

I looked at Norton. His shoulders indeed were squeezing. And then
I looked back at Kevin. "Blind you are," Kevin said, "and blind you
shall be." And I could see that, in a certain way, he might have been
right, not necessarily in his specific interpretation of Norton's communications, but in the generosity and plain reasonableness of his noting
the possibility of meaningfulness.

The narratives of the world are numberless, wrote the French semioti-
cian Roland Barthes (1977). In languages spoken or written, in images
fixed or moving, in gestures, motions, myths and legends, in movies and
theater performances, in paintings and stained-glass windows, in complex
orchestral compositions and in the simplest, most plaintive ancient melodies – in every age, in every place, in every society, there is no people without the impulse to tell. So plentiful are the forms of narrative, Barthes
wrote, it is as though almost "any material were fit to receive man's stories" (Barthes, 1977, p. 79). And so it is for our patients. Their meanings
are not limited to what words can express. They speak to us in a multiplicity of ways, some more readily accessible than others, some stunning in
their grotesqueness, some perhaps disgusting or acutely disturbing. But
each needing and deserving of our attention and engagement.

To become a psychiatric nurse means to embrace this perplexing
diversity of forms and to listen, respectfully, to what might be harbored
there. Instead of hurrying to contain a patient's bizarre presentations –
packaging violence, or aggressive preaching, or foreign-body ingestion, for example, in boxes labeled "symptoms" or "behaviors" needing
merely to be managed – this approach calls us to engage these presentations as actual ideas, as the suggestions of a story that wants to rise to
the surface of tell-ability. It is normal and natural, of course, to find
some behaviors frightening and some stories appalling and deeply dis-
quieting. But if we subject our emotional responses to the scrutiny of
thoughtful reflection, they may become, potentially, a source of knowledge, discovery, and richer, more respectful understanding.

Lingering inside a problem – "feeling it"

Nursing culture is a culture of efficiency. We pride ourselves on being "goal-directed" and "solution-focused." On action plans that strive toward specified aims. We identify a problem, list its operational objectives, execute plan elements, and document the achievements or failures to achieve stated aims, and so on. Knowing in advance what exactly we're aiming for, we are able to check our work. This is the kind of logic than enables self-assessment and high standards. It is the basis for accountability. But gestural bridging calls for a slightly different kind of logic. It is a logic of letting go. It asks not only that we strive toward a specified aim, but also – every so often – that we refrain from striving. This is the third principle embodied in the interventions described here: that we allow the mind to venture and stray sometimes from the instrumental logic of objectives-based planning and thinking.

Looking back at the story about Sara, we might remember that our approach did not start with a psychiatric diagnosis and follow down a list of associated goals and measurable objectives, as nursing interventions generally and rightfully do. Rather, it began with a simple turn of phrase – overheard in an ordinary conversation during wound dressing. In the small answer to a small question about where a swallowed item had lodged, we stumbled, suddenly and unexpectedly, on the suggestion of an inner configuration of thought. A door opened into consciousness. And from that small gateway, we were able to imagine a new form of interpersonal contact.

In Joe's case, medications and conventional treatment approaches hadn't proven effective over months of work. Empathic listening had been painful for anyone who tried it. But an unpleasant sensation – a feeling of being pushed around – registered itself in the body of an exhausted and aggravated nurse whose mind, near sleep, scanned its own repository of physical memory and found, in that personal past, an echo of some present theme. With Donald, many weeks of misery coalesced one morning into a passing observation made by a mother about teenagers – a fleeting comment that registered instantly as a collective gasp of the familiar. In Aaron's situation, it was simple body ache – our awareness of stuck-ness, of an inchoate grasping for order through rigid pacing – which gave sensible form to the idea that we needed, somehow, to change the tune. Who among us, after all, has not paced in frustration and found solace in the act of turning on the radio? We saw the singular moment, in the experience with Valerie, when the physical act of grabbing a doll rendered suddenly visible the common-sense understanding that an object held outside might refer in some way to the objects held inside. That structures might be erected outside to enable reference to the structures locked inside.

Some information sits for years at the margins of self-awareness. But it isn't lost. We've all had the experience of an image popping up suddenly, a sense that dawns all at once. Passing someone in a hallway, for example, calls up the resonating awareness of tobacco smell on an old friend's breath. Hearing a melody emanating from a passing car, we summon the face of an old school classmate who sang so beautifully on the park bench under the corner oak. These are not necessarily mere passing sensations. Rather, in some cases, they are amenable to be put to use. None of the ideas in this book could have been derived from a diagnostic manual or followed logically from conventional nursing-care objectives. Rather, they were generated by reference and association, by the wandering of meanings in the body.

To linger inside an idea is to allow ourselves to feel for its echoes, to note the contours it evokes in our own pool of memory and thought. This mode of arriving at an intervention is not the traditional professional mode of the nurse, though it is well known in art and, of course, in psychoanalysis, where transference and counter-transference are regarded as a primary source of information and treatment is expected to require an investment of utmost patience over periods of many years. To be open to the more distant sources of understanding is to access and make available, in our work, more of ourselves than is required by conventional approaches to therapeutic communication. It is to behave as the artist behaves – and to respond as the artist responds to the pulls and tugs of symbol and suggestion. It is to harness what has sometimes been called an *aesthetic attitude* – an innate human capacity, as I have argued here, inscribed in our earliest engagement in play and communication.

Appreciating the ordinary simplicity of a suddenly good idea

Which brings us to the fourth principle, about appreciating the suddenly illuminating clarity of a good idea. Many decades ago, I learned about the chemist Dmitri Mendeleev, who sought desperately to grasp the nature of matter. At the time Mendeleev worked, in the middle of the 19th century, chemistry and physics were a hodge-podge of disconnected facts and discoveries. No framework yet existed for explaining or tying together their basic principles – for answering questions about why, for example, there seemed to be classes of substances and materials which behaved similarly under particular conditions of temperature and pressure. So driven and perplexed was Mendeleev, so emotionally encumbered, it is said, that he made himself a deck of cards – and he printed on each card the name of a chemical substance and all its known attributes and properties. He'd spread the cards on a table and play, for hours, a kind of solitaire game, arranging and rearranging to see if any pattern might reveal its secrets. In the end, it was the game itself which ignited the legendary flash of recognition: sitting at a table with his cards one afternoon, Mendeleev invented what we now know as the Periodic Table – the fundamental organizing principle of modern chemistry.

All of us, from time to time, experience a sudden flip in our perceptions of things – a flash moment, so to speak, that shifts our vision and generates connections between elements which become, forever onward, inseparable in our minds. Here was the ordinary and familiar thing – the game of sorting cards into grid-like configurations of columns and rows – sparking the shock of recognition, the moment of singular coherence when diverse aspects of understanding coalesce into a resolute whole, binding themselves by the instrument of an effective metaphor. So it is for the insights which come to us about our patients. They arrive, at times, with a sudden and bracing simplicity.

Professional training and credentials give order and discipline to our thinking. But they can't make us good nurses. Care plans are important, since practices grounded in reasoned judgment have a greater chance of hitting the mark than choices made hastily and without evidence or previous trial. But they don't offer much guidance in our struggles with patients who have not responded to conventional treatments. An ideological commitment to caring is also important, as our work would be impossible without it. And it is crucial, of course, to understand the treatment norms connected to specific diagnoses, since interventions randomly targeted are pointless and, worse, potentially harmful. But, as the stories in this book illustrate, some of what nurses know derives not from any of these, but, rather, from an everyday capacity for imagination to meander across the sense modalities and wait for a moment when pieces might fall into place.

This is the "vision" which enables the blind, figuratively, to see, and the parent to sense naturally how to speak, in the gestural language of a warm embrace, to her infant's outstretched arms. It is the fundamental ability of thought to make itself felt, to announce its presence across the face of the body. It is the same innate human proclivity which transformed sounds, for Joe, into the sensation of physical boundaries, and dollhouse furniture, for Valerie, into spoken words. It forms the metaphoric basis of literature and art, as we have seen previously.

No DSM guides were referenced in the encounters described here. No list was made of symptom-management objectives derived from the patient's history of illness. Rather, in every case, an idea was born when a certain configuration of experience suddenly bound itself to something familiar in our own felt memory. Educational psychologist Jerome Bruner once noted that "a good representation is like a release from bondage" (Bruner, 1979, p. 26) – it has a clear somatic effect. After you've wrestled intensely with a problem, there is relief in the sudden materializing of a solution: something new appears, and we feel, clearly, that a burden has been lifted. So, too, for the encounters here between patient and nurse. Sometimes it is the simplest, ordinary thing which can be most clarifying and satisfying.

The body as an instrument of thought

Which brings us to the fifth principle: that the body itself is an instrument not only of feeling but of thought. It is a source of judgment. This is something we grasp tacitly – as when, faced with a choice, we ask "what does your gut say?" or, confronting a decision, we assess that "it feels right" or "seems like a good fit." This is a concept well known in the arts. The creation of a poem, a painting, or a melody depends upon the artist's ability to attend to highly nuanced qualitative relationships in a medium, as Elliot Eisner has written (2002). In music, the medium is sound; in the visual arts, it is form; in dance, it is movement. And so on. The artist working in each of these media must attend to properties and potentials specific to that medium and to the work as it unfolds, making moment-by-moment judgments by consulting somatic experience, asking "how does this image feel now, at this moment?" "Does it hang together?" "Does it satisfy?" These questions do not yield to recipe and algorithm, as Eisner has suggested. They are questions only the body can answer.

But while the artist is perhaps the exemplar, the paradigm, of an "aesthetic" approach, he or she is by no means its sole practitioner. Artistic activity is a form of everyday inquiry, as the philosopher John Dewey once wrote (Dewey, 1980), and all of us consult our bodies constantly in thinking through experience (Lakoff & Turner, 1989). Nursing theorist Peggy Chinn has referred to the turn to body consultation as the "artistic moment" in a nursing encounter (Chinn, 1994, p. 36) and noted that it differs from the more commonplace "empathic" understandings more conventionally associated with our profession. In each of the situations described in this book, in each case where metaphorical reasoning opened a door to more effective communication, we can see that the body figured as a component and active agent of meaning-making – it was a means of reaching out to the patient to ask and answer new questions.

Release and restraint – the role of self-discipline

Which brings us to the sixth core principle: about the interplay of feeling and thinking – of impulse and restraint. My patient Clement had recently been moved to a supervised apartment. The expansion of community placement options such as this answers decades of earlier failed attempts to deinstitutionalize the chronically mentally ill. I felt a sense of moral duty, both to Clement and to the reform movement his apartment represented. I wanted this to work. I wanted Clement to have independence and autonomy, to secure the same freedoms and rights for himself, despite his illness, as are expected for everyone else. So, every two weeks, as part of an outreach team, I checked on him – delivering his oral medications, administering his decanoate injections, ferrying him to the grocery store, and inspecting his cabinets and countertops for evidence of any relapse into heroin and alcohol. But every time I looked, the pantry was bare. Not a crumb to be seen.

I had taught Clement to make a budget, to list healthy foods and find them on the supermarket shelves, to switch the stove on and off, to wash dishes with soap, to order grocery delivery, and so on. But the dumpster at the back of the nearby Panda Wok restaurant remained, despite all my work, his primary source of food. I felt awful. I stepped up the frequency of my visits. I reassured him about my caring presence and availability. I promised persistence and began routinely checking his weight and vital signs and asking about nausea, vomiting, and breaks in the skin. I bought him fruit-and-vegetable smoothies, which weren't cheap, hoping to inspire some interest in alternatives to greasy Chinese food. I feared he might succumb to food poisoning, develop hypertension, cut himself on broken glass or, worse, be bitten by a rat. But nothing changed, the weeks passed, and I escalated into an alarm state as I documented in my progress notes the ongoing reiteration of life-skills teaching.

Then winter neared, leaves fell from the bushes, and aspects of Clement's life, previously obscured to me, suddenly revealed themselves. Across the street, in an abandoned factory lot piled with litter and filthy box-spring mattresses, Clement had been setting out foil trays of discarded restaurant food. I could see them now under the bushes as I pulled to the edge of the sidewalk in my company car, scattering mangy cats in many directions. Clement was dining outside, and he was dining with the strays. When I asked him, he confirmed it. In his choices about meals, Clement had effectively anointed himself the head of a kind of household – populating an intimate personal universe of whining felines over whom he presided, now, as provider and caretaker. A complicated and intellectually challenging story was telling itself under the bare branches of weedy *Ailanthus* in this little corner of the city: here was my patient's encounter, cast in the metaphor of cat food, with questions about giving and receiving, belonging and commanding, companionship and solitude, generosity and obligation. I had been diminishing this rich human struggle with my fixed assumptions about Clement's need for my compassion and for the kind of nursing care I had been giving him. Now, I had to think harder, and feel more deeply, about what might be done to enable this young man to sustain himself in the community setting, especially as cold weather loomed.

This is the sixth lesson: that empathy calls out for accuracy, feeling calls out for thinking. Warmth, compassion, and perseverance, the traditional nursing values, are a source of pride for our profession, and emotional connection is a key to good nursing. But the impulse to feel strongly and the desire to act compassionately call out, as well, for the taming discipline of reason and thoughtful reflection, for a commitment to restraint and precise targeting in the kind of care we perceive our patients to need. The approach described here asks that we take responsibility not just to *give* care, but also to *take care*. That is, to *be careful* – and to make sure that our feelings of concern, forceful though they might be, do not become possessive or territorial – do not obliterate the patient's world of ideas by folding it into our own professional narrative about nursing empathy and love.

Humility in an interdisciplinary context

Which brings us to the seventh principle: humility. By this I mean an openness to professional criticism, scrutiny, and reflection in the context of interdisciplinary work. The interventions described in this book were not first attempts at clinical engagement. Rather, they were measures of desperation, aimed at reaching very ill patients – those at the very far reaches of the illness spectrum – who had not responded to other forms of invitation to the treatment alliance. It needs to be remembered that the patients in every case, regardless of the setting, were taking medications, among relatively consistent clinical and support personnel, within structured case management routines, inside a framework of collaboration, supervision, and commitment to professional standards of care. Every patient eventually met, at least some time, with a wide circle of clinicians – a circle which included, in most cases, psychologists, psychiatrists, art and music therapists, social workers, addiction counselors, and so on – and drew from resources belonging not just to nursing but to the wider milieu. No nurse worked alone, and no nursing intervention can be understood apart from this context.

Nursing theory, in general, tends to claim far-reaching results for our work, and much of our professional literature describes what are taken to be fundamental and sweeping life changes in patients following relatively brief interpersonal encounters (Birnbaum, 2015). These claims no doubt hold true in many cases, and most of us can describe personal experiences which seem to bear them out. But they project, as well, our own deeply held desires to derive meaning from our work, feel efficacious in the face of human suffering, and claim a place for ourselves among the clinical disciplines. More realistically, as the stories here demonstrate, nurses might claim for ourselves something perhaps less grand but nonetheless crucial for our patients and for the work of our clinical teams. Bridging interventions are a unique nursing contribution not because they are the whole of treatment, transformative or curative in and of themselves, or because they are the end of treatment, solving a problem once and for all, but, rather, because they unlock a door – they open a transitional space in which patients can begin communicating with others. They enable other forms of therapeutically rich relationships to be launched.

Many of the clinical relationships which benefitted our patients were enabled to begin, in large part, as a direct result of the initial "bridging" work which nurses performed and which transitioned the patient into readiness for treatment. In this sense, "bridging" acknowledges that nursing, however unique in what it offers and contributes, is bound in a tight and mutually nurturing symbiosis with the work of other clinical disciplines. We tend to forget this sometimes, and collaborative teamwork, with some exceptions, is not yet built into the curriculum of most programs where nurses are trained.

There are dangers inherent in any approach which is creative and new, and nurses who find themselves motivated or inspired by the stories here will need to remain keenly aware of the potential for crossing personal and professional boundaries – for example, favoring some patients over others because we "like" the feeling of metaphoric engagement, or avoiding some patients because we cannot find a means of connecting to them, or badgering patients with game or activity ideas which aren't really sensitive or in tune with their needs in the moment. All of us know that patients are fragile, and that great harm can be done if we lose sight of the subtle ways our own private motivations and personal projections might embed themselves in our work. All the more so for the interventions described here, since they emerge from deeply personal, idiosyncratic responses to patients' symptoms and behaviors. Being creative does not mean losing humility and professional rigor. Quite the contrary, it requires a redoubling of the commitment to scrutiny and critique and a willingness to admit when an intervention seems self-serving or not to be going in the right direction. The benefit of more conventional care planning is that it protects patients from ideas which have not been fully thought through. Engaging in a new approach means taking a risk of being wrong. Rigorous self-reflection is the crucial starting point for any nurse who is interested in drawing on personal aesthetic sensibilities in the course of working with patients. Collaborating with other nurses and also with colleagues from other clinical disciplines forces us to subject our ideas to the test of shareability and collective review. It serves as a check on the potential for unrestrained experimentation and abuse of personal power.

Note

1 Portions of this chapter have appeared previously in Birnbaum, S. (2015). Freud still matters to nursing: a response to Sandra P. Thomas. *Issues in Mental Health Nursing* 36, 1017–1018. Reprinted by permission of Taylor & Francis.

References

Arieti, S. (1976). *Creativity: The magic synthesis*. New York, NY: Basic Books.

Barthes, R. (1977). *Image music text*. New York, NY: Hill and Wang.

Birnbaum, S. (2015). Freud still matters to nursing: a response to Sandra P. Thomas. *Issues in Mental Health Nursing* 36, 1017–1018.

Borbely, A. (2008). Metaphor in psychoanalysis. In R. Gibbs (Ed.), *The Cambridge handbook of metaphor and thought* (pp. 412–424). Cambridge: Cambridge University Press.

Bruner, J. (1979). *On knowing: Essays for the left hand*. Cambridge, MA: Harvard University Press.

Chinn, P.L. (1994). Developing a method for aesthetic knowing in nursing. In P.L. Chinn & J. Watson (Eds.), *Art and aesthetics in nursing* (pp. 19–40). New York, NY: National League for Nursing.

Dewey, J. (1980). *Art as experience*. New York, NY: Perigee Books.

Eisner, E.W. (1996). *Cognition and curriculum reconsidered* (2nd ed.). London: Paul Chapman Publishing.

Eisner, E.W. (2002). *The arts and the creation of mind*. New Haven, CT: Yale University Press.

Gibbs, R.W., Jr. (1994). *The poetics of mind: Figurative thought, language, and understanding*. New York, NY: Cambridge University Press.

Johnson, M. (1987). *The body in the mind: The bodily basis of meaning, imagination, and reason.* Chicago: University of Chicago Press.

Lakoff, G. & Turner, M. (1989). *More than cool reason: A field guide to poetic metaphor.* Chicago, IL: University of Chicago Press.

Modell, A. (2003). *Imagination and the meaningful brain.* Cambridge, MA: MIT Press.

Nightingale, F. (1859). *Notes on nursing: What it is, what it is not.* New York, NY: D. Appleton. Retrieved from https://www.digital.library.upenn.edu/women/nightingale/nursing.html

Rothenberg, A. (1988). *The creative process of psychotherapy.* New York, NY: W.W. Norton.

8 Conclusion

Millions of people come into contact with the mental health system every year, and many thousands wind up in the institutional system of care. Institutionalization can be a stultifying and frightening experience, involving physical and social isolation, loss of autonomy, and further disruption of already damaged life routines. When we take the nursing oath, we accept for ourselves a moral obligation to humanize what is inhumane in this situation and this system and to engage wholly in the work of restoring patients' access to maximal independence, safety, dignity, and self-regulation, even when they have not responded to previous attempts at engagement or treatment – and even when their outward behavior challenges and troubles us deeply. This book is an effort in that direction. It describes a form of therapeutic communication which has not been theorized previously in psychiatric nursing but which seems to hold promise as a means for engaging acutely ill institutionalized patients who have not responded to more conventional therapeutic approaches.

I have called this method the "gestural bridge," and I have given examples of how it was deployed to engage patients at times when they were particularly difficult to "reach" clinically. A gestural bridge can be said to represent an instance of what some cognitive linguists have called "conceptual metaphor" (Lakoff & Johnson, 1999). It is a way of taking a complex, abstract idea and giving it a form, without using words, by mapping it on to commonplace, readily accessible body-based schemas of experience and understanding. The idea receives a tentative, ad hoc representation in the form of a game or physical activity, rather than in conventional language.

In each situation described here, a patient was violent, aggressive, withdrawn, bizarre, or unready or unwilling for other reasons to participate in formal talk-based therapies or group programs. An activity was developed. It called for many of the traditional nursing competencies – caring, compassion, composure, patience, perseverance, and so on. But it

contained little in the way of conventional therapeutic language and format. Words of encouragement were not spoken. Absent were the usual
overt offers of empathy or support, the acknowledgment and the validation, the praises for good effort. Feelings were neither identified nor
talked about, and conscious insight was not a goal for the patients. There
was no specific care plan and no list of objectives read off from a psychiatric diagnosis. Rather, the aim was simple engagement, and the activity
looked more like a game than like conventional psychiatric nursing.

Appearing to be game-like or play-like, however, did not make the
activity frivolous or unserious. On the contrary, each of the interventions described in this book was structured in a specific and deliberate
way. It linked to something personally significant to the patient – casting
in the structure of its gestures and motions a theme the patient seemed
to be holding inside. It invited the patient to encounter an idea in a
wordless, sensory vocabulary that was familiar and non-threatening.
But it provided the nurse, at the same time, with a means to point to
new directions for feeling and thought. Straddling what is private in one
person and what could be shared in common with another, the activity
set in motion, between patient and nurse, a simple organizing image, a
metaphor, which enabled the patient to begin experiencing a problem in
a new way and to create what philosopher Paul Ricoeur has called new
"frameworks of connection" (Ricoeur, 1977).

By reconfiguring the stream of sensory and mental experience, even in a
small way, the games and activities described here effected a shift in what
philosophers and psychoanalysts, after Freud, have sometimes called the
"representability" or "figurability" of an idea (Castoriades, 2007; Botella
& Botella, 2005, 2013). At a time in a patient's life when he or she is unable to articulate or give voice to complex feelings or needs, this approach
offers the ultra-gentle nudge of a transitional dialect, an initiation into language – without quite being language itself. It begins the process of tearing
what might be say-able from what has not been said previously.

Let us review what happened in each of the examples offered here.
With Sara, games and activities were developed which suggested in
multiple small but repeating ways the separation of inside from outside. These activities "spoke" to her, without words, about borders
and boundaries. With Joe, a listening game activated themes of space
and place, suggesting that a sense of enveloping safety and belonging
is attainable and might be built by multiple means. With Donald, our
activities played on themes of yearning for entry and exit, of wanting to
take in and break out – allowing him to have these as a mental experience
before mastering a language for expressing them in words. With Valerie,
we developed activities which provided an external, concrete structure, a

vocabulary of shape and form which substituted for conventional words but pointed to the possibility of narrative-making. With Aaron, finally, our activities engaged themes of order, rhythm, and reciprocity; they were a way of reminding him about something he was missing.

In none of the encounters described here did the patient need to verbalize conscious understanding. There was no discussion about the mental associations which may or may not have been triggered during the course of engaging in the activity or game, about the movement of meanings across sensory modalities, or even about the feeling of having been cared for. Might we have talked to Donald directly, for example, about his yearning to break free from confinement? Or sat down with Sara to consider, together, her struggles with objects that had perforated her bowels? Of course not. Such conversations would have led nowhere. They might actually have been damaging, since the patients showed clearly that they were not ready for talk of this type. Rather, in each case, the behavioral response itself was the measure of the activity's effectiveness. We saw, in Aaron, the calming effect of rigorously ordered music, and in Joe, a dawning sense of comfort and belonging, the feeling of being surrounded by a personal space. We saw, in Donald, the cessation of violence and a new willingness to engage with clinical programming. In Sara, we could measure a reduction in self-harming behaviors, as with Valerie we witnessed a remarkable narrative emergence. In none of these situations, however, did we need to talk to the patients directly about what was happening. Writer Albert Rothenberg has noted that to try describing a metaphor in literal terms is to strip it of some of its power, deprive it of some of its vitality (Rothenberg, 1988). So, too, for the kind of play involved in a gestural bridge.

Gestural bridging harnesses the imaginative tools associated more often with poets and artists than with conventional nursing-care planning and understandings of patient care needs. It represents a form of aesthetically grounded therapeutic communication which has links to play therapy with children and with some of the themes which figure centrally in psychoanalytic approaches to treatment. For the most part, our professional has relegated poetry and art to the periphery – cast these as decorative and enriching, good for patients and perhaps an aspect of professional self-care – but not really central to our everyday professional work. The approach described here, on the contrary, restores the aesthetic to a central place in nursing.

In *Listening to Patients*, their book on phenomenological approaches to patient care, Thomas and Pollio (2002) suggest that thoughtful nursing grows not out of pre-conceived and computer-printable care plans but, rather, from an attunement to individual subjectivity and personal meanings in the patient's experience of illness. There have been multiple calls in recent years for a revival of the "aesthetic" in nursing practice – for creative approaches rooted in the "embodied experience" of nursing in real situations (Chinn & Kramer, 2014; Chinn & Watson, 1994; Hartrick, 2002; Hartrick Doane and Varcoe, 2013). Kagan, Smith, and Chinn (2014), along these lines, have emphasized the importance of commitment to the liberation of personal agency in the nurse–patient encounter. Gestural bridging is a metaphoric process of therapeutic communication which exemplifies these ideals as it connects psychiatric nursing to some of the foundational principles of other psychotherapeutic disciplines.

Nurses are particularly suited to developing interventions of this type because of our rich and unique access to patients. We spend more time with patients than do any other kind of clinician, which means we have more of a chance to get to know them – provided we make the most of it. We see patients in everyday situations rather than in scheduled "sessions," which means we develop an intimate understanding of their personal habits, rhythms, and responses in "real time." We engage with their bodies directly, in ways that bring us information unavailable to others in the clinical setting. For the most part, we are not bound to manualized treatment protocols and are free to respond to patients as situations and context demand. We could and should be making far better use of this special access to knowledge than is currently the norm.

Advocacy in a changing policy context

We are living in an era of fiscal restraint and widespread public- and private-sector downsizing. Policymakers and healthcare administrators promise a commitment to patient recovery and to high-quality mental healthcare. But cost-cutting measures continue to result in significant adverse changes in the staffing and task structures of many psychiatric treatment settings, eroding clinicians' capacity to do the intensive, collaborative, interdisciplinary work that professional duty demands and that patients deserve. In both the public and the private sectors, we see almost the same story: as a result of these changes, it is becoming increasingly difficult for nurses to do the kind of creative, thoughtful nursing we want and are trained to do. In this context, our future is bound with that of our patients. Advocating for them – for the most vulnerable, the most challenging and, often, the most publicly despised – we advocate for our own professional integrity and capacity. It is incumbent on us to take up this effort – to work for a robust, adequately financed, appropriately staffed and integrated system of care that ensures patients' access to creative and thoughtful treatment and maximizes their chances of getting out – and staying out – of restrictive institutional settings. I can only hope that this book contributes to making a case in that area.

If you are a nursing student or a new psychiatric nurse, you most likely have not realized yet the full scope of the personal and professional challenges you will face on the job. Little in your training can prepare you for the disturbing, often heart-rending, and sometimes frightening situations you will encounter, or for the complexities and frustrations of interdisciplinary clinical work. Under immense strain, you'll have to maintain a commitment to unwavering civility and intellectual curiosity and an attitude of utmost respect for your patients and their capacity and creativity. Apply yourself to this challenge.

References

Botella, C. & Botella, S. (2005). *The work of psychic figurability: Mental states without representation.* New York, NY: Routledge.

Botella, C., & Botella, S. (2013). Psychic figurability and unrepresented states. In H. Levine, G. Reed, & D. Scarfone (Eds.), *Unrepresented states and the construction of meaning: Clinical and theoretical contributions* (pp. 95–121). London: Karnac.

Castoriades, C. (2007). *Figures of the thinkable.* Stanford, CA: Stanford University Press.

Chinn, P., & Kramer, M. (2014). *Knowledge development in nursing: Theory and process* (9th ed.). New York, NY: Elsevier Mosby.

Chinn, P. & Watson, J. (Eds.). (1994). *Art and aesthetics in nursing.* New York, NY: National League for Nursing.

Hartrick, G. (2002). Transcending the limits of method: cultivating creativity in nursing. *Research and Theory for Nursing Practice* 16(1), 53–62.

Hartrick Doane, G. & Varcoe, C. (2013). *How to nurse: Relational inquiry with individuals and family in changing health and healthcare contexts.* New York, NY: Wolters Kluwer.

Kagan, P.N., Smith, M.C., & Chinn, P.L. (2014). *Philosophies and practices of emancipatory nursing: Social justice as praxis.* New York, NY: Routledge: Taylor & Francis.

Lakoff, G. & Johnson, M. (1999). *Philosophy in the flesh: The embodied mind and its challenge to Western thought.* New York, NY: Basic Books.

Ricoeur, P. (2012). *The rule of metaphor: Multidisciplinary studies of the creation of meaning in language.* Toronto, Ont.: University of Toronto Press.

Rothenberg, A. (1988). *The creative process of psychotherapy.* New York, NY: W.W. Norton.

Thomas, S.P., & Pollio, H.R. (2002). *Listening to patients: A phenomenological approach to nursing research and practice.* New York, NY: Springer.

Index

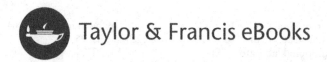

Taylor & Francis eBooks

Helping you to choose the right eBooks for your Library

Add Routledge titles to your library's digital collection today. Taylor and Francis ebooks contains over 50,000 titles in the Humanities, Social Sciences, Behavioural Sciences, Built Environment and Law.

Choose from a range of subject packages or create your own!

Benefits for you

>> Free MARC records
>> COUNTER-compliant usage statistics
>> Flexible purchase and pricing options
>> All titles DRM-free.

Benefits for your user

>> Off-site, anytime access via Athens or referring URL
>> Print or copy pages or chapters
>> Full content search
>> Bookmark, highlight and annotate text
>> Access to thousands of pages of quality research at the click of a button.

REQUEST YOUR **FREE** INSTITUTIONAL TRIAL TODAY

Free Trials Available
We offer free trials to qualifying academic, corporate and government customers.

eCollections – Choose from over 30 subject eCollections, including:

Archaeology	Language Learning
Architecture	Law
Asian Studies	Literature
Business & Management	Media & Communication
Classical Studies	Middle East Studies
Construction	Music
Creative & Media Arts	Philosophy
Criminology & Criminal Justice	Planning
Economics	Politics
Education	Psychology & Mental Health
Energy	Religion
Engineering	Security
English Language & Linguistics	Social Work
Environment & Sustainability	Sociology
Geography	Sport
Health Studies	Theatre & Performance
History	Tourism, Hospitality & Events

For more information, pricing enquiries or to order a free trial, please contact your local sales team:
www.tandfebooks.com/page/sales

Routledge
Taylor & Francis Group

The home of
Routledge books

www.tandfebooks.com

Printed in the United States
by Baker & Taylor Publisher Services

Printed in the United States
by Baker & Taylor Publisher Services